The **COMPLETE** Step-by-Step

DIABETIC
COOKBOOK

Developed by the Research Nutritionist of the
General Clinical Research Center, School of Medicine,
and the Registered Dietitians of the
Department of Food and Nutrition Services,
University Hospital, University of Alabama at Birmingham

Compiled and edited by Anne C. Cain, M.S., M.P.H., R.D.

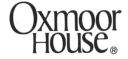
Oxmoor
House®

ISBN: 0-8487-3051-8
Printed in China
First printed in 1995

Editor-in-Chief: Nancy Fitzpatrick Wyatt
Executive Editor: Katherine M. Eakin
Art Director: Cynthia Rose Cooper
Copy Chief: Allison Long Lowery

The Complete Step•by•Step Diabetic Cookbook

Editor: Anne Chappell Cain, M.S., M.P.H., R.D.
Copy Editor: Cecilia C. Robinson
Editorial Assistant: Stacey Geary
Senior Production Designer: Larry Hunter
Director of Production: Phillip Lee
Production Manager: Theresa L. Beste
Production Assistant: Faye Porter Bonner
Publishing Systems Administrator: Rick Tucker

Contributors:
Recipe and Nutritional Analysis Consultant: Betty E. Darnell, M.S., R.D.,
        Director of Nutrition, General Clinical Research Center, University
        Hospital, University of Alabama at Birmingham
Photographer: Howard L. Puckett
Photo Stylist: Ashley J. Wyatt
Food Stylist: Julie Christopher

Cover: *Polynesian Beef* Kebabs *(page 139)*

To order additional publications, call 1-800-765-6400.

For more books to enrich your life, visit **oxmoorhouse.com**

Contents

INTRODUCTION

Here's a book that will make it easier to plan meals for you and your family. Though it's designed especially to help people with diabetes or those who cook for them, the recipes and meal planning techniques feature principles that apply to everyone who is concerned about healthy eating.

If you've used the *Cookbook for Diabetics and Their Families* or the *All-New Cookbook for Diabetics and Their Families* (Copyrights 1984 and 1988 by Oxmoor House, Inc.), the recipes on the following pages will be familiar to you. We've combined the best of the two previously published books in this updated, easy-to-follow edition. Flip through the pages of *The Complete Step·by·Step Diabetic Cookbook* and you'll find:

- Over 300 recipes, many of them family favorites with familiar, on-hand ingredients and simple cooking procedures

- Sugar-free, low-fat recipes developed and tested by registered dietitians at the University of Alabama at Birmingham

- Diabetic exchange values for every recipe (people following other meal plans with an exchange system will find this helpful, too)

- Exchange Lists from the *Exchange Lists for Meal Planning* formulated by The American Dietetic Association and the American Diabetes Association

- Nutrient values of each serving of every recipe including calories, carbohydrate, protein, fat, fiber, sodium, and cholesterol

- Step-by-step recipe procedures for every recipe

Diet is only part of the prescription for controlling blood sugar. Insulin, exercise, and meal schedule are all essential factors in the control of your diabetes. You and your health care team can work together to develop a treatment plan tailored to fit your lifestyle. Because diet plans, as well as insulin and medication requirements, are so individualized, this book simply offers you good recipes as a framework for meal planning. We recommend that you discuss your specific meal plan with your physician and a registered dietitian (R.D.).

These recipes will help you provide your family with healthy meals that don't single out a different plate for the person with diabetes. That's important–eating good food with people you love is something no one should miss!

The Editors

Eating Smart

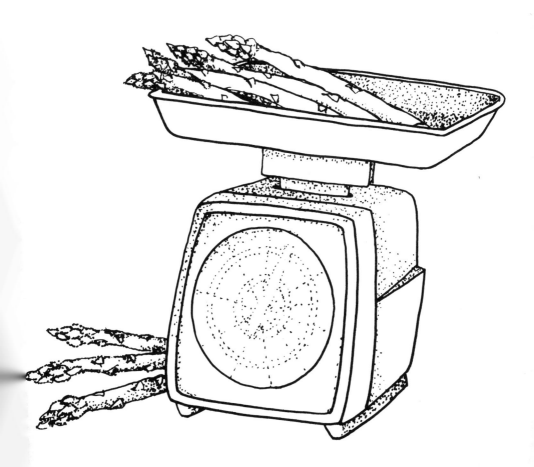

GUIDELINES FOR EATING SMART

We know that what we eat affects how we feel, how we look, and how we perform—today and tomorrow.

No one knows this better than people with diabetes. But a rigid diet is not the answer for most people; the answer is to *eat smart*. This means eating according to the basics of good nutrition that provide a foundation for good health.

You may be surprised to learn that what's nutritionally good for a diabetic person is nutritionally good for everyone else, too. And *nutritious* can be *delicious*. Our recipes prove it!

Recommended Dietary Guidelines

The third edition of the U.S. Dietary Guidelines for Americans provides a framework for healthy eating. These seven guidelines encourage variety, balance, and moderation, and offer a simplified approach for eating smart.

1. Eat a variety of foods.

If you are following a diabetic meal plan, you are already putting the first guideline into practice. No single food can supply all the nutrients you need. But by eating a variety of foods, you usually can supply your body with all the basic nutrients, including vitamins and minerals.

2. Maintain a healthy body weight.

A healthy weight is defined by how much of your weight is fat, where that body fat is located, and whether you have weight-related medical problems. See the height-weight chart below for suggested healthy weights. (The weight chart does not give different weights for men and women because the weight ranges given for each height are intended to take into account gender, frame size, and muscle mass.)

Suggested Weights for Adults

Height (without shoes)	Weight in Pounds (without clothes)	
	19 to 34 years	35 years and over
5'0"	97-128	108-138
5'1"	101-132	111-143
5'2"	104-137	115-148
5'3"	107-141	119-152
5'4"	111-146	122-157
5'5"	114-150	126-162
5'6"	118-155	130-167
5'7"	121-160	134-172
5'8"	125-164	138-178
5'9"	129-169	142-183
5'10"	132-174	146-188
5'11"	136-179	151-194
6'0"	140-184	155-199
6'1"	144-189	159-205
6'2"	148-195	164-210
6'3"	152-200	168-216
6'4"	156-205	173-222
6'5"	160-211	177-228
6'6"	164-216	182-234

3. Choose a diet low in fat, saturated fat, and cholesterol.

Keep your total fat intake to no more than 30% of total daily calories.

- Saturated fat should provide less than 10% of your total daily calories.
- Substitute polyunsaturated fats, especially monounsaturated fats, for saturated fats whenever possible.
- Limit dietary cholesterol intake to less than 300 milligrams a day.

4. Choose a diet with plenty of vegetables, fruits, and grain products.

These are the foods that provide carbohydrate in your diet which should make up at least one-half of the calories you consume daily.

5. Use sugars only in moderation.

Sugar substitutes may be used in the diet management of people with diabetes and people who are trying to lose weight.

Sugar substitutes do not have the same properties as sucrose (table sugar), but they do give foods a sweet taste. Although some substitutes contain calories, in most cases they're used in such small quantities that they don't add much to total caloric intake. The chart on page 354 shows you how to substitute alternative sweeteners for sugar in your favorite recipes.

6. Use salt and sodium only in moderation.

Salt and sodium may contribute to your risk of high blood pressure. If you are on a sodium-restricted diet, note the sodium content of recipes and decrease the added salt, if necessary.

7. If you drink alcoholic beverages, do so in moderation.

Alcohol affects the way insulin acts in your body and affects your blood sugar. Alcoholic beverages also contribute calories to your diet. Check with your physician and registered dietitian if you wish to include an alcoholic beverage in your meal plan.

MEAL PLANNING

Eating smart begins at the planning stage when you're deciding what to buy and how to prepare it. When you're changing your eating habits, remember that gradual changes are best. The following suggestions for buying and preparing foods will help you make smart choices.

SHOPPING: KNOW WHAT'S ON THE LABEL

Read the labels of products before you buy. The information on the **ingredient label** and the **Nutrition Facts** panel that now appears on most foods will help you make wise food choices.

An ingredient label must appear on all processed foods that contain more than one ingredient. It should list all ingredients in descending order by weight. Unfortunately, it's impossible to determine the percentage of each ingredient from this list. You need to look at the Nutrition Facts panel to determine the amount of sugar and fat in a product. Under new labeling laws, a Nutrition Facts panel must be displayed on almost all processed foods. See the label below for an example of the nutrition information that must appear on the new food labels.

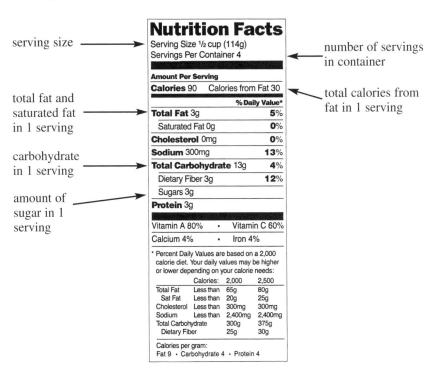

serving size →

total fat and saturated fat in 1 serving →

carbohydrate in 1 serving →

amount of sugar in 1 serving →

number of servings in container ←

total calories from fat in 1 serving

Nutrition Facts

Serving Size ½ cup (114g)
Servings Per Container 4

Amount Per Serving

Calories 90   Calories from Fat 30

	% Daily Value*
Total Fat 3g	5%
Saturated Fat 0g	0%
Cholesterol 0mg	0%
Sodium 300mg	13%
Total Carbohydrate 13g	4%
Dietary Fiber 3g	12%
Sugars 3g	
Protein 3g	

Vitamin A 80%	•	Vitamin C 60%
Calcium 4%	•	Iron 4%

* Percent Daily Values are based on a 2,000 calorie diet. Your daily values may be higher or lower depending on your calorie needs:

		Calories:	2,000	2,500
Total Fat	Less than		65g	80g
Sat Fat	Less than		20g	25g
Cholesterol	Less than		300mg	300mg
Sodium	Less than		2,400mg	2,400mg
Total Carbohydrate			300g	375g
Dietary Fiber			25g	30g

Calories per gram:
Fat 9 • Carbohydrate 4 • Protein 4

SUGAR: WHAT'S IN A NAME?

To find out if a food product contains sugar, check the label for any of the following terms:

Brown Sugar–a soft sugar in which crystals are covered by a film of refined dark syrup

Carbohydrate–a nutrient made up of sugars and starches

Corn Sugar–a sugar made by the breakdown of cornstarch

Corn Syrup–a syrup containing several different sugars that is obtained by the partial breakdown of cornstarch

Dextrin–a sugar formed by the partial breakdown of starch

Dextrose–another name for sugar

Fructose–the simple sugar found in fruit, juices, and honey

Galactose–a simple sugar found in lactose (milk sugar)

Honey–a sweet, thick material made in the honey sac of various bees

Invert Sugar–a combination of sugars found in fruit

Lactose–the sugar found in milk

Levulose–another name for fruit sugar

Maltose–a crystalline sugar formed by the breakdown of starch

Mannitol–a sugar alcohol

Maple Sugar–a syrup made by concentrating the sap of the sugar maple

Molasses–the thick syrup separated from raw sugar in the manufacturing process of sugar

Sorbitol–a sugar alcohol

Sorghum–a syrup from the juice of the sorghum grain grown mainly for its sweet juice

Starch–a powdery complex chain of sugars; for example, cornstarch

Sucrose–another name for table sugar

Sugar–a carbohydrate, including the monosaccharides: fructose, galactose, and glucose—and the disaccharides: sucrose, maltose, and lactose

Xylitol–a sugar alcohol

Xylose–a wood sugar found in corn cobs, straw, bran woodgum, and the bran of seeds, cherries, pears, peaches, and plums

Many "sugar-free" products, especially candies and cookies, are sweetened with sugar alcohols such as sorbitol, mannitol, and xylitol. Use products with sugar alcohols in limited amounts because they can cause diarrhea, and they still have calories and fat.

JUST A SPOONFUL OF SUGAR SUBSTITUTE

Many sugar substitutes have been developed for use as a sweetening agent for people with diabetes and for those trying to lose weight. Recipes in this cookbook that call for sugar substitutes were tested with either Sweet N' Low® or Sweet-10® liquid sugar substitute.

Sugar substitutes do not have the same properties as sucrose (table sugar) but do give foods a sweet taste; in fact, they are intensely sweet. Although some contain calories, in most cases substitutes are used in such small quantities that they do not significantly contribute to caloric intake.

When using sugar substitutes, remember that they do not have the same cooking properties as table sugar for brownness, lightness, and tenderness in foods. Some sugar substitutes undergo chemical changes when heated, causing a bitter taste in the finished product. Other sugar substitutes are not recommended for use in baking.

You may want to try several brands and amounts of sugar substitutes to see which type of sweetener you prefer. Several brands with substitution equivalents for sugar are listed in the sugar substitution chart on page 354. Always read the manufacturer's instructions regarding recommended use of specific sweeteners.

See Sugar Substitutions on page 354

PREPARATION: MAKE IT LIGHT

Try to use food preparation methods that help to decrease sugar and fat. The following cooking techniques apply to weight-reduction diets as well as to diabetic diets. As you look at the recipes, notice these methods and ingredients.

- Meats are baked or broiled rather than fried.
- Vegetables are steamed, boiled, or sautéed in a nonstick skillet.
- Desserts are sweetened with sugar substitutes or fruit juices instead of sugar.
- Pasta and rice are cooked with no added salt or fat.
- Vegetable cooking spray is used instead of shortening or butter to coat pans and baking dishes.

PERFECT PORTIONS

After properly cooking foods, the next step is measuring the appropriate serving size. Only by measuring will you get the correct amount of calories and carbohydrates in your diet. The Exchange Lists that begin on page 16 tell you what amount of a particular food is equal to one serving. Use the following guidelines to measure your food.

- Measure the food as you would eat it—after it is cooked, without the bone, skin, or inedible parts.
- Weigh meats on small kitchen scales. Fruit also may be weighed on these scales.
- Measure most vegetables, cereals, and fruit with dry-measure cups. If a serving calls for ½ cup, the food should be level with the top of the measuring cup.
- Use liquid-measure cups for fluids such as milk or fruit juices.
- Use teaspoons or tablespoons for foods such as margarine, mayonnaise, peanut butter, salad dressings, and sour cream. The food should be level and not heaped on the spoon.

HERBS AND SPICE AND EVERYTHING NICE

Add flavor, aroma, and variety to recipes by seasoning foods with herbs and spices instead of fat and salt. To substitute dried herbs for fresh, use approximately one-third of the fresh amount. Herbs and spices are free foods and don't have to be counted in your meal plan. (See the Free Foods List on page 28.)

MEALS AWAY FROM HOME

For most Americans, eating out is now a routine instead of a luxury. Don't let an on-the-go schedule keep you from following your meal plan. Use the following tips for food selection when you're not in your own kitchen.

DINING OUT

Many restaurants are now featuring healthier fare on their menus to meet consumer demand. Be sure to ask questions about the fat or sugar content of an item if it is not clear from the menu description. Use the following list below to help you make healthy choices when eating out.

Appetizers
- Order "free" foods such as clear broth, bouillon, consommé, or fresh vegetables such as carrot and celery sticks.
- Count fresh fruit and fruit juices, soups, shrimp cocktail, and crackers in your meal plan.

Meat, Poultry, and Fish
- Select broiled, baked, roasted, and grilled meats, fish, or poultry. Request that gravies and sauces be omitted or served on the side.
- Avoid casseroles and fried items. If you select a breaded or fried item, count the breading and fat in your meal plan, or remove the breading.

Salads
- Select vegetable and fresh fruit salads.
- Request that the salad dressing be served on the side.
- Use lemon juice or vinegar as a "free" salad dressing.
- Avoid coleslaw, canned fruit, and gelatin salads.
- Count starchy salads such as pasta salad, potato salad, and three-bean salad in your meal plan.

Breads
- Choose plain bread, rolls, toast, muffins, crackers, and breadsticks; be sure to watch the serving sizes.

- Remember that some breads, such as biscuits, cornbread, pan-cakes, and hush puppies, contain fat and should be counted as a starch plus a fat exchange.

Vegetables

- Select raw, stewed, steamed, baked, and grilled vegetables.
- Avoid fried vegetables and vegetables in a cream or cheese sauce.

Starchy Side Dishes

- Select baked, steamed, and boiled potatoes, rice, and plain pasta.
- Check the size of baked potatoes; a potato approximately 2 inches in diameter equals 1 Starch Exchange.
- Request that margarine and sour cream be served on the side.
- Avoid fried items and those served in a cream sauce.

Desserts

- Select fresh fruit or fruit juices.
- Choose plain ice cream, sherbet, frozen yogurt, and plain cake such as sponge or angel food cake.

FAST FOOD

Most fast-food restaurants offer items that will fit into your meal plan. Avoid those that are obviously high in sugar and fat, such as milk shakes, fruit pies, sundaes, and regular soft drinks. See pages 32–33 for a list of Fast Food Exchanges, or ask for a list at the restaurant.

BROWN BAGGING

Your meal plan can be adapted to include foods that are easily portable.

- Make sandwiches with thin-sliced meats and cheeses or leftover meats. Add variety by using different breads–pumpernickel, rye, sourdough, white, and whole wheat. Also try sandwiches with bagels, rolls, and pita bread.
- Pack leftover casseroles, stews, and soups in wide-mouth thermoses or pack in airtight containers and reheat in a micro-wave oven.
- Include canned vegetable or fruit juices, or pack raw carrot and celery sticks, a fresh tomato, or fresh fruit.

USING THE EXCHANGE LISTS

The six Exchange Lists (food groups) below were developed to help people with diabetes plan their meals. The individual diet plan prescribed by your physician and/or registered dietitian indicates the number of servings from each food group that you should eat at each meal and for snacks.

All the foods within a group contain about the same amount of nutrients and calories per serving, which means that one serving of a food from the starch list may be exchanged (or substituted) for one serving of any other item in the starch list. The chart below shows the amount of nutrients and number of calories in one serving from each food group.

Exchange List	Calories	Carbohydrate (grams)	Protein (grams)	Fat (grams)
Starch/Bread	80	15	3	trace
Meat				
Lean	55	–	7	3
Medium-Fat	75	–	7	5
High-Fat	100	–	7	8
Vegetable	25	5	2	–
Fruit	60	15	–	–
Milk				
Skim	90	12	8	trace
Low-Fat	120	12	8	5
Whole	150	12	8	8
Fat	45	–	–	5

The Exchange Lists beginning on page 16 are the basis of a meal planning system designed by a committee of the American Diabetes Association and The American Dietetic Association. (Copyright 1989 by the American Diabetes Association, Inc., and The American Dietetic Association.) While designed primarily for people with diabetes and others who must follow specific diets, the Exchange Lists are based on principles of good nutrition that apply to everyone.

The American Diabetes Association has many publications to help you live better with diabetes. For more information or to order a free publications catalog, call the American Diabetes Association at 1-800-232-3472, extension 355 or 363.

Starch List

Each item in this list contains approximately 15 grams of carbohydrate, 3 grams of protein, a trace of fat, and 80 calories. Foods that contain 3 or more grams of fiber per serving are identified with a * symbol.

You can choose your starch exchanges from any of the items on this list. If you want to eat a starch food that is not on this list, follow these general rules:

½ cup of cereal, grain, or pasta equals one serving (1 starch exchange)

1 ounce of a bread product equals one serving (1 starch exchange)

Your registered dietitian can help you be more exact.

CEREALS, GRAINS, AND PASTA

*Bran cereals, concentrated	
(such as Bran Buds®, All Bran®)	⅓ cup
*Bran cereals, flaked	½ cup
Bulgur (cooked)	½ cup
Cooked cereals	½ cup
Cornmeal (dry)	2½ tablespoons
Grapenuts	3 tablespoons
Grits (cooked)	½ cup
Other ready-to-eat unsweetened cereals	¾ cup
Pasta (cooked)	½ cup
Puffed cereal	1½ cups
Rice, white or brown (cooked)	⅓ cup
Shredded wheat	½ cup
*Wheat germ	3 tablespoons

DRIED BEANS, PEAS, AND LENTILS

*Beans and peas (cooked),	
such as kidney, white, split, black-eyed	⅓ cup
*Lentils (cooked)	⅓ cup
*Baked beans	¼ cup

STARCHY VEGETABLES

*Corn	½ cup
*Corn on cob (6-inch ear)	1
*Lima beans	½ cup
*Peas, green (canned or frozen)	½ cup
*Plantain	½ cup
Potato, baked	1 small (3 ounces)
Potato, mashed	½ cup
*Squash, winter (acorn, butternut)	1 cup
Yam, sweet potato, plain	⅓ cup

BREAD

Bagel	½ (1 ounce)
Bread sticks, crisp, (4 x ½ inch)	2 (⅔ ounce)
Croutons, low-fat	1 cup
English muffin	½
Frankfurter or hamburger bun	½ (1 ounce)
Pita (6-inch diameter)	½
Plain roll, small	1 (1 ounce)
Raisin, unfrosted	1 slice (1 ounce)
Rye, pumpernickel	1 slice (1 ounce)
Tortilla, corn (6-inch diameter)	1
White (including French, Italian)	1 slice (1 ounce)
Whole wheat	1 slice (1 ounce)

CRACKERS AND SNACKS

Animal crackers	8
Graham crackers (2½-inch square)	3
Matzoh	¾ ounce
Melba toast	5 slices
Oyster crackers	24
Popcorn (popped, no fat added)	3 cups
Pretzels	¾ ounce
*Rye crisp (2 x 3½ inches)	4
Saltine-type crackers	6
*Whole wheat crackers, no fat added (crisp breads, such as Finn®, Kavli®, Wasa®)	2–4 slices (¾ ounce)

STARCH FOODS PREPARED WITH FAT

Count each item in this list as 1 Starch Exchange plus 1 Fat Exchange

Biscuit (2½-inch diameter)	1
Chow mein noodles	½ cup
Cornbread (2-inch cube)	1
Cracker, round butter-type	6
French fried potatoes	
(2 to 3½ inches long)	10
Muffin, plain, small	1
Pancake (4-inch diameter)	2
Stuffing, bread (prepared)	¼ cup
Taco shell (6-inch diameter)	1
Waffle (4½-inch square)	1
*Whole-wheat crackers, fat added	4–6 (1 ounce)
(such as Triscuit®)	

Count each item in this list as 1 Starch Exchange plus 2 Fat Exchanges

Corn chips	1 ounce
Potato chips	1 ounce
Tortilla chips	1 ounce

Meat List

Each serving of meat and meat substitutes on this list contains about 7 grams of protein. The amount of fat and number of calories vary depending on the type of meat or meat substitute you choose. The meat list is divided into three sections based on the amount of fat and calories. One ounce (1 Meat Exchange) of each includes:

	Calories	Carbohydrate (grams)	Protein (grams)	Fat (grams)
Lean	55	0	7	3
Medium-Fat	75	0	7	5
High-Fat	100	0	7	8

Try to replace high-fat meats with lean and medium-fat meats, poultry, and fish. This will help decrease your fat intake. The items from the high-fat group are high in saturated fat, cholesterol, and calories. You should limit your choices from the high-fat group to three per week.

Meat and meat substitutes that have 400 milligrams or more of sodium per serving are indicated with a • symbol. A •• symbol means that two servings of this food will provide 400 milligrams or more of sodium.

LEAN MEAT AND SUBSTITUTES
Count each item in this list as 1 Meat Exchange

Beef:	USDA Select or Choice grades of lean beef such as round, sirloin, and flank steak; tenderloin; •chipped beef	1 ounce
Pork:	Lean pork such as fresh ham; canned, cured, or •boiled ham; •Canadian bacon; tenderloin	1 ounce
Veal:	All cuts are lean except for veal cutlets (ground or cubed). Examples of lean veal are chops and roasts.	1 ounce
Poultry:	Chicken, turkey, Cornish hen (without skin)	1 ounce
Fish:	All fresh and frozen fish	1 ounce
	Crab, lobster, scallops, shrimp, clams (fresh or canned in water)	2 ounces
	Oysters	6 medium
	••Tuna (canned in water)	¼ cup

Meat List *(continued)*

	••Herring (uncreamed or smoked)	1 ounce
	Sardines (canned)	2 medium
Game:	Venison, rabbit, squirrel	1 ounce
	Pheasant, duck, goose (without skin)	1 ounce
Cheese:	••Cottage cheese	¼ cup
	Parmesan, grated	2 tablespoons
	•Low-fat cheeses (less than 55 calories per ounce)	1 ounce
Other:	•Low-fat luncheon meat	1½ ounces
	Egg whites	3 whites
	Egg substitutes (less than 55 calories per ½ cup)	½ cup

MEDIUM-FAT MEAT AND SUBSTITUTES

Count each item in this list as 1 Meat plus ½ Fat Exchange

Beef:	Most beef products fall into this category. Examples: all ground beef, roast (rib, chuck, rump), steak (cubed, Porterhouse, T-bone), and meat loaf.	1 ounce
Pork:	Most pork products fall into this category. Examples: chops, loin roast, Boston butt, and cutlets.	1 ounce
Lamb:	Most lamb products fall into this category. Example: chops, leg, and roast.	1 ounce
Veal:	Cutlet (ground or cubed, unbreaded)	1 ounce
Poultry:	Chicken (with skin), domestic duck or goose (well drained of fat), ground turkey	1 ounce
Fish:	••Tuna (canned in oil and drained)	¼ cup
	••Salmon (canned)	¼ cup
Cheese:	Part-skim ricotta	¼ cup
	Part-skim mozzarella	1 ounce
	•Low-fat cheeses (56–80 calories per ounce)	1 ounce
Other:	••Reduced-fat luncheon meat	1 ounce
	Eggs (high-cholesterol; limit, 3 per week)	1
	Egg substitutes (56–80 calories per ¼ cup)	¼ cup
	Tofu (2½ x 2¾ x 1 inch)	4 ounces
	Liver, heart, kidney, sweetbreads (high-cholesterol)	1 ounce

HIGH-FAT MEAT AND SUBSTITUTES
Count each item in this list as 1 meat plus 1 Fat Exchange

Beef:	Most USDA Prime cuts of beef, such as ribs, ••corned beef	1 ounce
Pork:	Spareribs, ground pork, •pork sausage (patty or link)	1 ounce
Lamb:	Patties (ground lamb)	1 ounce
Fish:	Any fried fish product	1 ounce
Cheese:	All regular cheeses such as •American, •blue, ••Cheddar, ••Monterey Jack, Swiss	1 ounce
Other:	•Luncheon meats such as bologna, salami, pimiento loaf	1 ounce
	•Sausage such as Polish, Italian smoked	1 ounce
	•Knockwurst	1 ounce
	••Bratwurst	1 ounce
	•Frankfurter (turkey or chicken) (10 per pound)	1 frank
	Peanut butter (contains unsaturated fat)	1 tablespoon

Count as 1 Meat plus 2 Fat Exchanges

•Frankfurter (beef, pork, or combination) (10 per pound)	1 frank

Vegetable List

Each vegetable serving on this list contains about 5 grams of carbohydrate, 2 grams of protein, and 25 calories. A serving of vegetables usually contains 2 to 3 grams of dietary fiber. Vegetables that contain 400 or more milligrams of sodium per serving are identified with a • symbol.

Unless otherwise noted, the following are the serving sizes for vegetables (1 Vegetable Exchange):

½ cup of cooked vegetables or vegetable juice
1 cup of raw vegetables

Artichoke (½ medium)
Asparagus
Beans (green, wax, Italian)
Bean sprouts
Beets
Broccoli
Brussels sprouts
Cabbage, cooked
Carrots
Cauliflower
Eggplant
Greens (collard, mustard, turnip)
Kohlrabi
Leeks

Mushrooms, cooked
Okra
Onions
Pea pods
Peppers (green)
Rutabaga
•Sauerkraut
Spinach, cooked
Summer squash
Tomato (one large)
•Tomato/vegetable juice
Turnips
Water chestnuts
Zucchini, cooked

Starchy vegetables such as corn, peas, and potatoes are found on the Starch List beginning on page 16. For free vegetables, see the Free Foods List on page 28.

Fruit List

Each item on this list contains about 15 grams of carbohydrate and 60 calories. Fresh, frozen, and dried fruit have about 2 grams of fiber per serving. Fruit that has 3 or more grams of fiber per serving has a * symbol. Fruit juices contain very little dietary fiber.

The carbohydrate and calorie content for a fruit serving are based on the usual serving of the most commonly eaten fruits. Unless otherwise noted, the following are the serving sizes for one fruit serving (1 Fruit Exchange):

½ cup of fresh fruit or fruit juice
¼ cup of dried fruit

FRESH, FROZEN, AND UNSWEETENED CANNED FRUIT

Apple, raw (2-inch diameter)	1
Applesauce, unsweetened	½ cup
Apricots, medium, raw	4
Apricots, canned	½ cup or 4 halves
Banana (9-inch)	½ banana
*Blackberries	¾ cup
*Blueberries	¾ cup
Cantaloupe (5-inch diameter)	⅓ cantaloupe
Cantaloupe, cubes	1 cup
Cherries, large, raw	12
Cherries, canned	½ cup
Figs, raw (2-inch diameter)	2
Fruit cocktail, canned	½ cup
Grapefruit, medium	½ grapefruit
Grapefruit, segments	¾ cup
Grapes, small	15
Honeydew melon, medium	⅛ melon
Kiwifruit, large	1 kiwifruit
Mandarin oranges	¾ cup
Mango, small	½ mango
*Nectarine (2½-inch diameter)	1
Orange (2½-inch diameter)	1
Papaya	1 cup
Peach (2¾-inch diameter)	1
Peaches, sliced, raw	¾ cup

Peaches, canned	½ cup or 2 halves
Pear, raw	½ large or 1 small
Pears, canned	½ cup or 2 halves
Persimmon, medium	2
Pineapple, raw	¾ cup
Pineapple, canned	⅓ cup
Plum, raw (2-inch diameter)	2
*Pomegranate	½ pomegranate
*Raspberries	1 cup
*Strawberries, whole	1¼ cups
*Tangerine (2½-inch diameter)	2
Watermelon, cubes	1¼ cups

DRIED FRUIT

*Apples	4 rings
*Apricots	7 halves
Dates, medium	2½
*Figs	1½
*Prunes, medium	3
Raisins	2 tablespoons

FRUIT JUICE

Apple juice/cider	½ cup
Cranberry juice cocktail	⅓ cup
Grapefruit juice	½ cup
Grape juice	⅓ cup
Orange juice	½ cup
Pineapple juice	½ cup
Prune juice	⅓ cup

Milk List

Each serving of milk or milk products on this list contains about 12 grams of carbohydrate and 8 grams of protein. The amount of fat in milk is measured in percent (%) of butterfat. The calories vary, depending on the kind of milk you choose. The list is divided into three sections based on the amount of fat and calories. One serving (1 Milk Exchange) of each of these includes the following:

	Calories	Carbohydrate (grams)	Protein (grams)	Fat (grams)
Skim/Very Low-Fat	90	12	8	trace
Low-Fat	120	12	8	5
Whole	150	12	8	8

SKIM AND VERY LOW-FAT MILK
Count each item in this list as 1 Milk Exchange

Skim milk	1 cup
½% milk	1 cup
1% milk	1 cup
Low-fat buttermilk	1 cup
Evaporated skim milk	½ cup
Dry nonfat milk	⅓ cup
Plain nonfat yogurt	8 ounces

LOW-FAT MILK
Count each item in this list as 1 Milk plus 1 Fat Exchange

2% milk	1 cup
Plain low-fat yogurt	8 ounces

WHOLE MILK
Count each item in this list as 1 Milk plus 2 Fat Exchanges

The whole milk group has much more fat per serving than the skim and low-fat groups. Whole milk has more than 3¼% butterfat. Try to limit your choices from the whole milk group as much as possible.

Whole milk	1 cup
Evaporated whole milk	½ cup
Whole plain yogurt	8 ounces

Fat List

Each serving on the fat list contains about 5 grams of fat and 45 calories. The foods on the fat list contain mostly fat, although some items may also contain a small amount of protein. All fats are high in calories and should be carefully measured. Modify your fat intake by eating unsaturated fats instead of saturated fats.

The sodium content of these foods varies widely. A • symbol means that one serving of the food contains 400 milligrams or more of sodium. A •• symbol means that two or more servings of the food will provide 400 milligrams or more or sodium.

UNSATURATED FATS

Avocado	⅛ medium
Margarine	1 teaspoon
••Margarine, diet	1 tablespoon
Mayonnaise	1 teaspoon
••Mayonnaise, reduced-calorie	1 tablespoon
Nuts and seeds:	
Almonds, dry roasted	6 whole
Cashews, dry roasted	1 tablespoon
Peanuts	20 small or 10 large
Pecans	2 whole
Walnuts	2 whole
Other nuts	1 tablespoon
Seeds, pine nuts, sunflower	
(without shells)	1 tablespoon
Pumpkin seeds	2 teaspoons
Oil (corn, cottonseed,	
safflower, soybean,	
sunflower, olive, peanut)	1 teaspoon
••Olives	10 small or 5 large
Salad dressing, mayonnaise-type	2 teaspoons
Salad dressing, mayonnaise-type,	
reduced-calorie	1 tablespoon
••Salad dressing (oil varieties)	1 tablespoon
•Salad dressing, reduced-calorie	2 tablespoons

(2 tablespoons low-calorie salad dressing is a free food)

SATURATED FATS

Butter	1 teaspoon
••Bacon	1 slice
Chitterlings	½ ounce
Coconut, shredded	2 tablespoons
Coffee whitener, liquid	2 tablespoons
Coffee whitener, powder	4 teaspoons
Cream (light, coffee, table)	2 tablespoons
Cream, sour	2 tablespoons
Cream (heavy, whipping)	1 tablespoon
Cream cheese	1 tablespoon
••Salt pork	¼ ounce

Free Foods List

A free food is any food or drink that contains less than 20 calories per serving. You can eat as much as you want of those items that have no serving size specified.

BEVERAGES

Bouillon or broth (fat-free)
Bouillon (low-sodium)
Carbonated drinks, sugar-free
Carbonated water
Club soda
Cocoa powder, unsweetened
   (1 tablespoon)

Coffee
Drink mixes, sugar-free
Tea
Tonic water, sugar-free

FRUIT

Cranberries, unsweetened (½ cup)
Lemon

Lime
Rhubarb, unsweetened (½ cup)

CONDIMENTS

Ketchup (1 tablespoon)
Horseradish
Mustard
Pickles, dill, unsweetened
Salad dressing, low-calorie
   (2 tablespoons)

Soy sauce
Taco sauce (3 tablespoons)
Vinegar
Worcestershire sauce

VEGETABLES
(raw, 1 cup)

Cabbage
Celery
Chinese cabbage
Cucumber
Green onions

Mushrooms
Peppers, hot
Radishes
Zucchini

SALAD GREENS

Endive
Escarole
Lettuce

Romaine
Spinach

SWEET SUBSTITUTES

Candy, hard, sugar-free (1 piece)
Gelatin, sugar-free
Gum, sugar-free
Jam/jelly, sugar-free (less than 20
   calories per 2 teaspoons)

Pancake syrup, sugar-free
   (1 to 2 tablespoons)
Sugar substitutes
Whipped topping (2 tablespoons)

MISCELLANEOUS

Vegetable cooking spray

SEASONINGS

All herbs, spices, and most seasonings are considered free foods. Try to avoid seasonings or spice blends such as apple pie spice that contain sugar.

Also be careful of how much sodium or salt you use. Seasonings such as seasoning salt, garlic salt, onion salt, and poultry seasoning all contain salt. Read the label, and choose those seasonings that do not contain sodium or salt. Use any of the seasonings below to enhance the flavors of your favorite foods.

Basil
Bay leaves
Caraway seeds
Cardamom
Celery seeds
Chili powder
Chives
Cinnamon
Cloves
Coriander
Cumin
Curry
Dillweed
Fennel
Flavoring extracts
   (vanilla, almond,
   walnut, peppermint,
   butter, lemon, etc.)
Garlic

Garlic powder
Ginger
Herb and spice blend,
   salt-free
Dried Italian seasoning
Lemon
Lemon juice
Lemon pepper
Mace
Marjoram
Mint
Nutmeg
Onion powder
Oregano
Paprika
Pepper
Pepper sauce, hot
Pimiento
Poultry seasoning

Rosemary
Saffron
Sage
Savory
Soy sauce, regular and
   low-sodium
Tarragon
Thyme
Turmeric
Wine, used in cooking
   ($\frac{1}{4}$ cup)
Worcestershire sauce,
   regular and
   low-sodium

Combination Foods

Much of the food we eat is mixed together in various combinations. These combination foods don't fit into only one exchange list. Below is a list of average values for some typical combination foods that will help you fit them into your meal plan. Foods that have 400 milligrams or more of sodium are indicated with a • symbol. Ask your registered dietitian for information about any other foods you'd like to eat. Many other publications available provide exchange values for combination foods. Check your library or local bookstore, or contact the American Diabetes Association at 1-800-232-3472.

Food	*Amount*	*Exchanges*
Casseroles, meat and starch (homemade)	1 cup	2 Starch 2 Medium-Fat Meat 1 Fat
•Cheese pizza, thin crust	¼ of 10" pizza	2 Starch 1 Medium-Fat Meat 1 Fat
•Chili with beans (commercial)	1 cup	2 Starch 2 Medium-Fat Meat 2 Fat
•Chow mein (without noodles or rice)	2 cups	1 Starch 2 Vegetable 2 Lean Meat
•Macaroni and cheese	1 cup	2 Starch 1 Medium-Fat Meat 2 Fat
•Spaghetti and meatballs (canned)	1 cup	2 Starch 1 Medium-Fat Meat 1 Fat

Sugar-free pudding (made with skim milk)	½ cup	1 Starch

Soups:

•Bean	1 cup	1 Starch 1 Vegetable 1 Lean Meat
•Chunky, all varieties	1 (10¾-ounce) can	1 Starch 1 Vegetable 1 Medium-Fat Meat
•Cream (made with water)	1 cup (8 ounces)	1 Starch 1 Fat
•Vegetable or broth	1 cup (8 ounces)	1 Starch

If beans are used as a meat substitute:

Dried beans, peas, lentils	1 cup (cooked)	2 Starch 1 Lean Meat

Fast Food Exchanges

Product	Serving Size	Exchanges
ARBY'S		
Roast Beef Sandwich	1	2 Starch, 2 Medium-Fat Meat, 1½ Fat
Beef and Cheddar Sandwich	1	3 Starch, 2½ Medium-Fat Meat, 2 Fat
Light Roast Turkey Deluxe Sandwich	1	2 Starch, 2 Lean Meat
Grilled Chicken Deluxe Sandwich	1	2½ Starch, 2½ Medium-Fat Meat, 1 Fat
BURGER KING		
Hamburger	1	2 Starch, 2 Medium-Fat Meat
Cheeseburger	1	2 Starch, 2 Medium-Fat Meat, 1 Fat
Whopper	1	3 Starch, 3 Medium-Fat Meat, 3 Fat
French Fries	1	3 Starch, 3 Fat
HARDEE'S		
Hamburger	1	2 Starch, 1 Medium-Fat Meat, 1 Fat
Cheeseburger	1	2 Starch, 1 Medium-Fat Meat, 2 Fat
Big Roast Beef Sandwich	1	2 Starch, 3 Medium-Fat Meat
Rise 'N' Shine Biscuit	1	2 Starch, 4 Fat
Sausage Biscuit	1	2 Starch, 1 High-Fat Meat, 4 Fat
McDONALD'S		
Hamburger	1	2 Starch, 1 Medium-Fat Meat, 1 Fat
Cheeseburger	1	2 Starch, 1½ Medium-Fat Meat, 1 Fat
Quarter Pounder	1	2 Starch, 3 Medium-Fat Meat, 1 Fat
Big Mac	1	3 Starch, 2½ Medium-Fat Meat, 2 Fat

Fillet-O-Fish	1	2½ Starch, 1 Medium-Fat Meat, 2 Fat
Egg McMuffin	1	2 Starch, 2 Medium-Fat Meat
Hash Brown Potatoes	1	1 Starch, 1 Fat
Chicken McNuggets	6 pieces	1 Starch, 2 Medium-Fat Meat, 1 Fat

KENTUCKY FRIED CHICKEN

Drumstick, original recipe	1	2 Medium-Fat Meat
Side Breast, original recipe	1	½ Starch, 2½ Medium-Fat Meat, ½ Fat
Drumstick, extra crispy	1	½ Starch, 2 Medium-Fat Meat, ½ Fat
Side Breast, extra crispy	1	1 Starch, 2 Medium-Fat Meat, 3½ Fat
Coleslaw	1	2 Vegetable, 1 Fat

PIZZA HUT
Thin 'N' Crispy Pizza

Pepperoni	1 slice, medium pizza	1 Starch, 1½ Medium-Fat Meat, 1 Fat
Supreme	1 slice, medium pizza	1 Starch, 2 Medium-Fat Meat, 1 Fat

Pan Pizza

Pepperoni	1 slice, medium pizza	2 Starch, 1 Medium-Fat Meat, 2 Fat
Supreme	1 slice, medium pizza	2 Starch, 1½ Medium-Fat Meat, 1 Fat

TACO BELL

Beef Burrito	1	2½ Starch, 2 Medium-Fat Meat, 1 Fat
Beefy Tostada	1	1½ Starch, 1½ Medium-Fat Meat, 2 Fat
Burrito Supreme	1	3 Starch, 1½ Medium-Fat Meat, 2 Fat
Taco	1	1 Starch, 2 Lean Meat

Printed with permission from *Fast Food Facts*, Marion J. Franz, M.S., R.D., C.D.E., International Diabetes Center, Minneapolis, Minnesota, 1994. All rights reserved.

Snacks

Most people on diabetic diets have snacks already calculated into their diet plans. Use your meal plan as your guide for the appropriate type and amount of food. Some ideas for snacks are listed below:

Cereal and skim milk
Cheese and crackers
Fresh fruit and low-fat cottage cheese
Graham crackers and skim milk
Ice cream, sugar-free
Peanut butter and crackers
Peanut butter and rice cakes
Popcorn, air-popped
Pretzels
Pudding, sugar-free
Sandwich
Vanilla wafers and skim milk
Yogurt, low-fat or nonfat
Frozen yogurt, sugar-free
Free foods (see list on page 28)

Food for Sick Days

Your diabetes may be harder to control when you have a cold or the flu and are not able to follow your meal plan. The following guidelines should help in your meal planning for these times. For other special instructions you may need to contact your physician.

- Continue to take your insulin or hypoglycemic agent as prescribed.

- Follow your meal plan as closely as possible. Eat only foods and liquids that you can digest easily, such as soups, crackers, cereals, juices, soft drinks, and soft fruit.

- Try to limit your foods to the starch, fruit, and milk groups. Omit foods from the meat, vegetable, and fat groups during the illness.

- Drink plenty of liquids, especially if fever, vomiting, or diarrhea is present. If you are following your regular meal pattern, your extra liquids should be noncaloric, such as water, sugar-free soft drinks, or other unsweetened liquids.

- If you cannot eat solid foods, try sweetened liquids, such as fruit juices, regular soft drinks, popsicles, regular fruit-flavored gelatin, and noncarbonated, low-sodium natural thirst quencher, to replace the carbohydrates in regular food. Consume these only in small amounts throughout the day.

- If you have problems chewing or swallowing (for example, after you have had dental work), try eating regular foods that have been processed in a blender. Remember to measure foods before you blend them.

Below is a list of foods suitable for sick days. Each item can be substituted for 15 grams of carbohydrate or 1 Starch or Fruit Exchange. Use these as advised by your physician.

Apple juice	½ cup
Applesauce	½ cup
Carbonated beverages	
(containing sugar)	¾ cup (6 ounces)
Cooked cereal	½ cup
Crackers, saltine-type	6
Custard, baked	½ cup
Gatorade®	1 cup
Ginger ale	¾ cup
Grape juice	⅓ cup
Jell-O® (regular)	½ cup
Popsicle® (3-ounce size)	1
Soups, broth-based	
(such as chicken noodle)	2 cups
Soups, cream	1 cup
Toast	1 slice
Yogurt, plain	1 cup

USING THE NUTRITIONAL ANALYSIS

A nutritional analysis for one serving of each recipe in this book appears below the recipe title and the exchange values. The nutritional analysis lists the portion size of one serving.

Nutrient values are listed in whole numbers. If a nutrient is analyzed to have a value of 0.5 or more, it is rounded up to a whole number. If it is found to be less than 0.5, then a trace amount of the nutrient is available. If a nutrient has no value in a recipe, 0 will be listed.

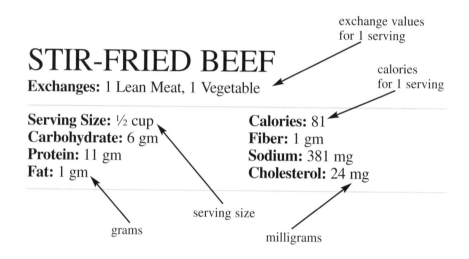

exchange values
for 1 serving

calories
for 1 serving

STIR-FRIED BEEF
Exchanges: 1 Lean Meat, 1 Vegetable

Serving Size: ½ cup
Carbohydrate: 6 gm
Protein: 11 gm
Fat: 1 gm

Calories: 81
Fiber: 1 gm
Sodium: 381 mg
Cholesterol: 24 mg

grams

serving size

milligrams

Beverages

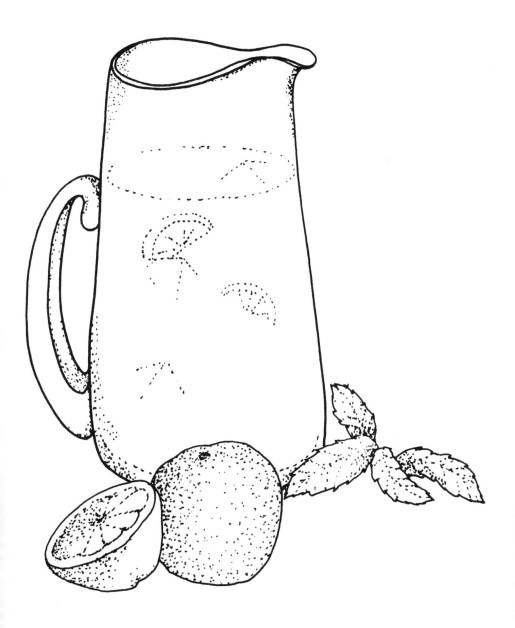

COCOA

Exchanges: 1 Skim Milk

Serving Size: 1 cup	**Calories:** 83
Carbohydrate: 13 gm	**Fiber:** 1 gm
Protein: 7 gm	**Sodium:** 252 mg
Fat: 1 gm	**Cholesterol:** 3 mg

INGREDIENTS:

2 tablespoons unsweetened cocoa
¼ teaspoon salt
1 cup water

3 cups skim milk
Sugar substitute to equal 8 teaspoons sugar*
1 teaspoon vanilla extract

STEPS IN PREPARATION:

1. Combine cocoa and salt in a small saucepan. Add water, and place over low heat or in top of a double boiler. Boil gently, stirring constantly, 2 minutes.
2. Add milk and sugar substitute. Bring to a boil, stirring constantly; remove from heat immediately.
3. Stir in vanilla, and serve warm.

Yield: 4 servings

*See the sugar substitution chart on page 354.

SPICED HOT TEA

Exchanges: Free

Serving Size: ⅔ cup
Carbohydrate: 2 gm
Protein: trace
Fat: trace

Calories: 6
Fiber: 0 gm
Sodium: 5 mg
Cholesterol: 0 mg

INGREDIENTS:

4 cups water
1 cinnamon stick
3 whole cloves
Dash of ground nutmeg

2 thin lemon slices with rind
2 thin orange slices with rind
3 or 4 regular-size tea bags,
  as desired

STEPS IN PREPARATION:

1. Combine first 6 ingredients in a heavy saucepan; simmer 10 minutes.
2. Add tea bags, and let steep to taste. Remove tea bags, cinnamon stick, and cloves, and serve warm.

Yield: 6 servings

Use cinnamon sticks for hot beverage stirrers or float thin lemon slices on top for garnish and eye appeal.

LOW-CALORIE SPICED TEA MIX

Exchanges: Free

Serving Size: 1 teaspoon	**Calories:** 7
Carbohydrate: 1 gm	**Fiber:** trace
Protein: trace	**Sodium:** 1 mg
Fat: trace	**Cholesterol:** 0 mg

INGREDIENTS:

¾ cup sugar-free iced tea mix

¼ cup plus 2 tablespoons sugar-free orange-flavored drink mix

¼ cup sugar-free lemonade-flavored drink mix

2 tablespoons ground cinnamon

1 teaspoon ground cloves

STEPS IN PREPARATION:

1. Combine all ingredients, stirring until blended. Store mixture in an airtight container.
2. For each serving, place 1 teaspoon mix in a mug. Add 1 cup hot water, stirring well. Serve warm.

Yield: 72 servings

LEMON-ORANGE TEA

Exchanges: Free

Serving Size: ¾ cup
Carbohydrate: 6 gm
Protein: trace
Fat: trace

Calories: 25
Fiber: trace
Sodium: 10 mg
Cholesterol: 0 mg

INGREDIENTS:

½ cup boiling water
2 regular-size tea bags
Sugar substitute to equal 2
tablespoons sugar*
1½ cups cold water
1 cup unsweetened orange
juice

2 tablespoons lemon juice
1 (12-ounce) can sugar-free
lemon-lime carbonated
beverage

STEPS IN PREPARATION:

1. Pour boiling water over tea bags. Cover and let stand 5 minutes. Remove and discard tea bags. Transfer tea mixture to a medium pitcher, and stir in sugar substitute.
2. Add cold water, orange juice, and lemon juice. Cover and chill at least 1 hour.
3. Just before serving, add lemon-lime beverage to tea mixture, stirring well. Serve over ice.

Yield: 6 servings

*See the sugar substitution chart on page 354.

FRESH LEMONADE OR LIMEADE

Exchanges: Free (up to 4 cups per day)

Serving Size: 1 cup	**Calories:** 14
Carbohydrate: 4 gm	**Fiber:** 0 gm
Protein: trace	**Sodium:** 8 mg
Fat: trace	**Cholesterol:** 0 mg

INGREDIENTS:

¼ cup fresh lemon or lime
  juice
Sugar substitute to equal 4
  teaspoons sugar*

1¾ cups cold water
Fresh mint leaves (optional)
Lemon or lime wedges
  (optional)

STEPS IN PREPARATION:

1. Combine juice and sugar substitute; add water, and stir well.
2. Serve over ice. If desired, garnish with mint leaves and lemon or lime wedges.

Yield: 2 servings

*See the sugar substitution chart on page 354.

APRICOT FIZZ

Exchanges: 1 Fruit

Serving Size: 1 cup
Carbohydrate: 18 gm
Protein: trace
Fat: trace

Calories: 72
Fiber: trace
Sodium: 15 mg
Cholesterol: 0 mg

INGREDIENTS:

3 cups unsweetened apricot juice, chilled

3 cups sugar-free ginger ale, chilled

1 tablespoon lemon juice

STEPS IN PREPARATION:

1. Combine all ingredients; stir well.
2. Pour into individual glasses, and serve immediately.

Yield: 6 servings

If unsweetened apricot juice is not available, you can use unsweetened apricot nectar. Or try unsweetened peach juice instead of apricot juice– 1 cup will still equal 1 Fruit Exchange.

CITRUS COOLER

Exchanges: 1 Fruit

Serving Size: 1 cup	**Calories:** 67
Carbohydrate: 16 gm	**Fiber:** trace
Protein: trace	**Sodium:** 2 mg
Fat: trace	**Cholesterol:** 0 mg

INGREDIENTS:

¾ cup boiling water
½ cup fresh mint leaves, coarsely chopped
4 cups sugar-free lemonade
1 cup unsweetened orange juice

1 cup unsweetened pineapple juice
¾ cup unsweetened grapefruit juice
Sugar substitute to equal ½ cup sugar*

STEPS IN PREPARATION:

1. Pour boiling water over mint leaves. Cover and let stand 5 to 15 minutes. Strain mixture, discarding mint leaves. Transfer mint-flavored water to a large pitcher.
2. Add lemonade and remaining ingredients, stirring until blended. Cover and chill 2 hours.

Yield: 7 servings

*See the sugar substitution chart on page 354.

CRAN-ORANGE PUNCH

Exchanges: 1 Fruit

Serving Size: ½ cup
Carbohydrate: 11 gm
Protein: trace
Fat: trace

Calories: 47
Fiber: 0 gm
Sodium: 7 mg
Cholesterol: 0 mg

INGREDIENTS:

1¼ cups reduced-calorie
  cranberry juice cocktail
Sugar substitute to equal ¼
  cup sugar*
1 (6-ounce) can frozen orange
  juice concentrate, thawed
  and undiluted

2 cups sugar-free lemon-lime
  carbonated beverage

STEPS IN PREPARATION:

1. Combine cranberry juice, sugar substitute, and orange juice concentrate in a large bowl; stir well, and chill.
2. Just before serving, add lemon-lime beverage to fruit juice mixture. Serve over crushed ice.

Yield: 8 servings

*See the sugar substitution chart on page 354.

HOLIDAY PUNCH

Exchanges: ½ Fruit

Serving Size: 1 cup	**Calories:** 21
Carbohydrate: 5 gm	**Fiber:** 0 gm
Protein: trace	**Sodium:** 17 mg
Fat: trace	**Cholesterol:** 0 mg

INGREDIENTS:

3½ cups sugar-free lemon-lime carbonated beverage
2½ cups reduced-calorie cranberry juice cocktail

2 tablespoons lemon juice

STEPS IN PREPARATION:

1. Combine all ingredients in a punch bowl or pitcher.
2. Serve over ice.

Yield: 6 servings

Regular cranberry juice cocktail contains about three times as much carbohydrate as reduced-calorie cranberry juice, but both have essentially the same amount of vitamin C.

TROPICAL FRUIT PUNCH

Exchanges: 1 Fruit

Serving Size: ½ cup
Carbohydrate: 12 gm
Protein: trace
Fat: trace

Calories: 47
Fiber: 0 gm
Sodium: 7 mg
Cholesterol: 0 mg

INGREDIENTS:

3 cups unsweetened
   pineapple juice
2 cups sugar-free lemon-lime
   carbonated beverage
½ cup unsweetened lime
   juice

Sugar substitute to equal ¼
   cup sugar*
2 teaspoons rum extract
Orange slices (optional)

STEPS IN PREPARATION:

1. Combine first 5 ingredients in a large pitcher; stir well.
2. Serve over ice, and garnish with orange slices, if desired.

Yield: 11 servings

*See the sugar substitution chart on page 354.

TROPICAL ICE

Exchanges: 1 Fruit

Serving Size: ½ cup
Carbohydrate: 13 gm
Protein: trace
Fat: trace

Calories: 53
Fiber: 1 gm
Sodium: 4 mg
Cholesterol: 0 mg

INGREDIENTS:

2½ cups unsweetened orange
  juice
2 cups mashed banana
Sugar substitute to equal 1
  cup sugar*
1 tablespoon lemon juice

1 (20-ounce) can crushed
  pineapple in juice, undrained
1 (32-ounce) bottle sugar-free
  ginger ale
12 fresh strawberries
  (optional)

STEPS IN PREPARATION:

1. Combine first 5 ingredients in a large pitcher; stir well. Freeze until firm.
2. To serve, let stand at room temperature until partially thawed. Place in a punch bowl, and break into chunks. Add ginger ale, and stir until chunks soften. Garnish with fresh strawberries, if desired.

Yield: 24 servings

*See the sugar substitution chart on page 354.

PINEAPPLE-PEACH SMOOTHIE

Exchanges: 1 Fruit, 1 Skim Milk

Serving Size: 1 cup	**Calories:** 144
Carbohydrate: 29 gm	**Fiber:** 1 gm
Protein: 8 gm	**Sodium:** 106 mg
Fat: trace	**Cholesterol:** 3 mg

INGREDIENTS:

½ cup canned pineapple chunks in juice, undrained
½ cup unsweetened pineapple juice
2 canned peach halves in water, drained and diced

1 cup plain nonfat yogurt
1 cup skim milk
Sugar substitute to equal 2 tablespoons sugar*

STEPS IN PREPARATION:

1. Combine first 3 ingredients in container of an electric blender or food processor; cover and process until pureed.
2. Add yogurt, milk, and sugar substitute; continue to process until smooth and thickened.
3. Pour into individual glasses, and serve immediately.

Yield: 3 servings

*See the sugar substitution chart on page 354.

CHOCOLATE-BANANA SHAKE

Exchanges: 1 Fruit, 1 Skim Milk

Serving Size: 1 cup	**Calories:** 129
Carbohydrate: 26 gm	**Fiber:** 1 gm
Protein: 7 gm	**Sodium:** 94 mg
Fat: trace	**Cholesterol:** 3 mg

INGREDIENTS:

2 cups skim milk

1 teaspoon unsweetened cocoa

1 medium banana, sliced

STEPS IN PREPARATION:

1. Combine all ingredients in container of an electric blender or food processor; cover and process until frothy.
2. Pour into individual glasses, and serve immediately.

Yield: 3 servings

ORANGE-YOGURT SHAKE

Exchanges: 1 Fruit, ½ Skim Milk

Serving Size: ½ cup
Carbohydrate: 18 gm
Protein: 5 gm
Fat: trace

Calories: 91
Fiber: trace
Sodium: 54 mg
Cholesterol: 2 mg

INGREDIENTS:

1 (6-ounce) can frozen orange
   juice concentrate, thawed
   and undiluted

1 cup skim milk
¾ cup plain nonfat yogurt

STEPS IN PREPARATION:

1. Combine all ingredients in container of an electric blender or food processor; cover and process until smooth.
2. Pour into individual glasses, and serve immediately.

Yield: 5 servings

Don't be confused by the amount of fat in yogurt. Low-fat yogurt contains 0.5 to 2 percent milkfat by weight; nonfat yogurt contains less than 0.5 percent milkfat. Both come in a variety of fruit flavors as well as plain.

STRAWBERRY-ORANGE SHAKE

Exchanges: 1 Skim Milk, ½ Fruit

Serving Size: 1 cup	**Calories:** 115
Carbohydrate: 18 gm	**Fiber:** trace
Protein: 9 gm	**Sodium:** 160 mg
Fat: 1 gm	**Cholesterol:** 5 mg

INGREDIENTS:

1½ cups skim milk
⅓ cup fresh strawberries
2 tablespoons unsweetened
   orange juice

Sugar substitute to equal 2
   tablespoons sugar*
½ cup nonfat buttermilk

STEPS IN PREPARATION:

1. Combine first 4 ingredients in container of an electric blender or food processor. Cover and process until strawberries are pureed and mixture is frothy.
2. Transfer mixture to a small pitcher. Stir in buttermilk.
3. Pour into individual glasses, and serve immediately.

Yield: 2 servings

*See the sugar substitution chart on page 354.

Breads and Cereals

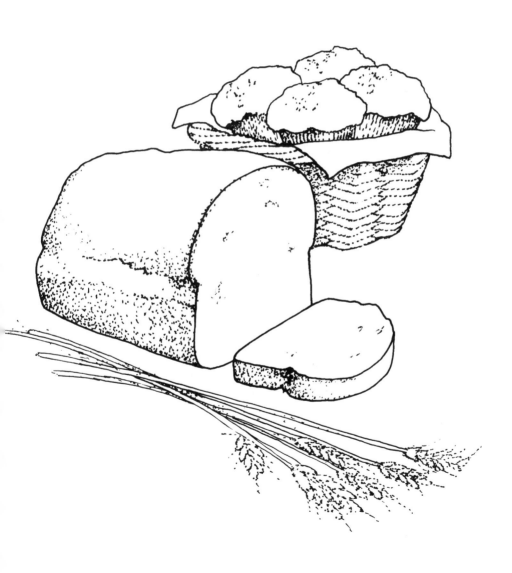

BISCUITS

Exchanges: 1 Starch, 1 Fat

Serving Size: 1 biscuit
Carbohydrate: 15 gm
Protein: 2 gm
Fat: 6 gm

Calories: 125
Fiber: 1 gm
Sodium: 129 mg
Cholesterol: 1 mg

INGREDIENTS:

1 package dry yeast
2 tablespoons warm water
  (105° to 115°)
2 cups nonfat buttermilk
5 cups all-purpose flour
1 tablespoon baking powder
1 teaspoon baking soda
1 teaspoon salt
Sugar substitute to equal
  ¼ cup sugar*
1 cup vegetable shortening

STEPS IN PREPARATION:

1. Combine yeast and warm water; let stand 5 minutes or until bubbly.
2. Add buttermilk to yeast mixture, and set aside.
3. Combine flour and next 4 ingredients in a large bowl; cut in short-ening with a pastry blender until mixture resembles coarse meal.
4. Add buttermilk mixture to flour mixture, stirring with a fork until dry ingredients are moistened.
5. Turn dough out on a floured surface, and knead lightly 3 or 4 times. Roll dough to ½-inch thickness; cut into 36 rounds with a 2-inch biscuit cutter, and place on ungreased baking sheets. Bake at 400° for 10 to 12 minutes or until golden.

Yield: 3 dozen biscuits

*See the sugar substitution chart on page 354.

MOM'S BISCUIT WEDGES

Exchanges: 1 Starch, 1 Fat

Serving Size: 1 wedge
Carbohydrate: 17 gm
Protein: 3 gm
Fat: 6 gm

Calories: 133
Fiber: 1 gm
Sodium: 268 mg
Cholesterol: trace

INGREDIENTS:

2 cups all-purpose flour
2½ teaspoons baking powder
½ teaspoon baking soda
Sugar substitute to equal 1
   tablespoon sugar*

¾ cup reduced-calorie
   margarine
¾ cup nonfat buttermilk

STEPS IN PREPARATION:

1. Combine first 4 ingredients in a medium bowl, stirring to blend. Cut in margarine with a pastry blender until mixture resembles coarse meal.
2. Add buttermilk, stirring just until dry ingredients are moistened.
3. Turn dough out onto a lightly floured surface, and knead 8 to 10 times. Divide dough into thirds. Gently shape each third into a ball; place 2 inches apart on an ungreased baking sheet.
4. Flatten each ball into a 1-inch-thick circle, and score each into four wedges. Bake at 400° for 10 to 15 minutes or until golden. Separate into wedges, and serve warm.

Yield: 1 dozen wedges

*See the sugar substitution chart on page 354.

APPLE MUFFINS

Exchanges: 1 Starch, ½ Fat

Serving Size: 1 muffin	**Calories:** 102
Carbohydrate: 17 gm	**Fiber:** 1 gm
Protein: 3 gm	**Sodium:** 226 mg
Fat: 3 gm	**Cholesterol:** 16 mg

INGREDIENTS:

1⅔ cups all-purpose flour
2½ teaspoons baking powder
½ teaspoon salt
Sugar substitute to equal 1
   tablespoon sugar*
1 teaspoon ground cinnamon
¼ teaspoon ground nutmeg

⅔ cup skim milk
¼ cup reduced-calorie
   margarine, melted
1 egg, lightly beaten
1 cup minced apple
Vegetable cooking spray

STEPS IN PREPARATION:

1. Combine first 6 ingredients in a medium bowl.
2. Combine milk, margarine, and egg; add egg mixture to dry ingredients, stirring just until dry ingredients are moistened. Fold in apple.
3. Spoon batter into nonstick muffin pans coated with cooking spray, filling two-thirds full. Bake at 400° for 25 minutes or until lightly browned.

Yield: 1 dozen muffins

*See the sugar substitution chart on page 354.

BRAN MUFFINS

Exchanges: 1 Starch, ½ Fat

Serving Size: 1 muffin
Carbohydrate: 17 gm
Protein: 3 gm
Fat: 3 gm

Calories: 102
Fiber: 2 gm
Sodium: 233 mg
Cholesterol: 16 mg

INGREDIENTS:

1 cup hot water
1 cup shreds of wheat bran
  cereal
½ cup reduced-calorie
  margarine
Liquid sugar substitute to
  equal 1 cup sugar*
2 cups nonfat buttermilk

2 eggs, lightly beaten
2½ cups all-purpose flour
2½ teaspoons baking soda
½ teaspoon salt
2 cups wheat bran flakes
  cereal
Vegetable cooking spray

STEPS IN PREPARATION:

1. Pour hot water over shreds of bran cereal; let stand at room temperature 10 minutes.
2. Cream margarine and sugar substitute in a large bowl. Add buttermilk, eggs, and soaked bran cereal, beating well at medium speed of an electric mixer.
3. Combine flour, soda, and salt; stir into creamed mixture. Fold in 2 cups bran flakes cereal.
4. Cover and store in refrigerator until ready to bake. (Batter can be stored in refrigerator up to 1 week.)
5. Spoon batter into muffin pans coated with cooking spray, filling two-thirds full. Bake at 400° for 15 minutes or until lightly browned.

Yield: 2 dozen muffins

*See the sugar substitution chart on page 354.

RAISIN-BRAN MUFFINS

Exchanges: 1 Starch, ½ Fat

Serving Size: 1 muffin
Carbohydrate: 14 gm
Protein: 3 gm
Fat: 3 gm

Calories: 85
Fiber: 2 gm
Sodium: 214 mg
Cholesterol: 16 mg

INGREDIENTS:

½ cup all-purpose flour
1 teaspoon baking soda
2 cups wheat bran cereal
1 cup nonfat buttermilk
¼ cup reduced-calorie
   margarine, melted

Liquid sugar substitute to
   equal ¼ cup sugar*
1 egg, lightly beaten
¼ cup plus 2 tablespoons
   raisins
Vegetable cooking spray

STEPS IN PREPARATION:

1. Combine flour and soda in a medium bowl; add bran cereal.
2. Combine buttermilk, margarine, sugar substitute, and egg; add to dry ingredients, stirring just until moistened. Fold in raisins.
3. Spoon batter into muffin pans coated with cooking spray, filling two-thirds full. Bake at 400° for 18 to 20 minutes or until lightly browned.

Yield: 1 dozen muffins

*See the sugar substitution chart on page 354.

Wheat bran cereal is a good source of insoluble fiber. Health experts encourage Americans to aim for a total fiber intake of 20 to 35 grams per day.

CORNMEAL MUFFINS

Exchanges: 1 Starch, ½ Fat

Serving Size: 1 muffin	**Calories:** 91
Carbohydrate: 16 gm	**Fiber:** 1 gm
Protein: 3 gm	**Sodium:** 220 mg
Fat: 2 gm	**Cholesterol:** 16 mg

INGREDIENTS:

1 cup yellow cornmeal
¾ cup all-purpose flour
1½ teaspoons baking powder
½ teaspoon baking soda
½ teaspoon salt
Sugar substitute to equal 1
  tablespoon sugar*

1 cup nonfat buttermilk
2 tablespoons reduced-calorie
  margarine, melted
1 egg, lightly beaten
Vegetable cooking spray

STEPS IN PREPARATION:

1. Combine first 6 ingredients in a medium bowl. Mix lightly with a fork.
2. Combine buttermilk, margarine, and egg; stir well. Add to cornmeal mixture. Stir well; then beat gently for 1 to 2 minutes.
3. Spoon batter into muffin pans coated with cooking spray, filling two-thirds full. Bake at 400° for 25 to 30 minutes or until lightly browned.

Yield: 1 dozen muffins

*See the sugar substitution chart on page 354.

OATMEAL-BLUEBERRY MUFFINS

Exchanges: 1 Starch, 1 Fat

Serving Size: 1 muffin
Carbohydrate: 22 gm
Protein: 5 gm
Fat: 6 gm

Calories: 160
Fiber: 2 gm
Sodium: 201 mg
Cholesterol: 16 mg

INGREDIENTS:

2 cups regular oats, uncooked
1 cup plus 2 tablespoons
  all-purpose flour
1 tablespoon baking powder
½ teaspoon salt
Sugar substitute to equal 2
  tablespoons sugar*

1 cup skim milk
¼ cup vegetable oil
1 egg
1 cup fresh blueberries
Vegetable cooking spray
1 teaspoon ground cinnamon

STEPS IN PREPARATION:

1. Combine first 5 ingredients in a medium bowl; make a well in center of mixture.
2. Combine milk, oil, and egg; add to dry ingredients, stirring just until dry ingredients are moistened. Fold in blueberries.
3. Spoon batter into muffin pans coated with cooking spray, filling two-thirds full.
4. Sprinkle cinnamon over muffins, and bake at 425° for 20 to 25 minutes or until lightly browned.

Yield: 1 dozen muffins

*See the sugar substitution chart on page 354.

TROPICAL MUFFINS

Exchanges: 1 Starch, 1 Fat

Serving Size: 1 muffin
Carbohydrate: 23 gm
Protein: 3 gm
Fat: 4 gm

Calories: 143
Fiber: 1 gm
Sodium: 237 mg
Cholesterol: 15 mg

INGREDIENTS:

1¾ cups all-purpose flour
2 teaspoons baking powder
¼ teaspoon baking soda
½ teaspoon salt
Sugar substitute to equal ¾ cup sugar*
¼ cup unsweetened shredded coconut
⅓ cup reduced-calorie margarine, melted

1 teaspoon grated orange rind
⅓ cup unsweetened orange juice
3 medium-size ripe bananas, mashed
1 egg, lightly beaten
Vegetable cooking spray

STEPS IN PREPARATION:

1. Combine first 5 ingredients in a large bowl; stir in coconut, and make a well in center of mixture.
2. Combine margarine, orange rind, orange juice, banana, and egg; add mixture to dry ingredients, stirring just until dry ingredients are moistened.
3. Spoon batter into muffin pans coated with cooking spray, filling two-thirds full. Bake at 375° for 25 to 30 minutes or until lightly browned.

Yield: 1 dozen muffins

*See the sugar substitution chart on page 354.

BANANA-APPLE BREAD

Exchanges: 1 Starch, 1 Fat

Serving Size: 1 (½-inch) slice
Carbohydrate: 21 gm
Protein: 3 gm
Fat: 4 gm

Calories: 123
Fiber: 1 gm
Sodium: 142 mg
Cholesterol: 23 mg

INGREDIENTS:

½ cup reduced-calorie
  margarine
Sugar substitute to equal 1 cup
  plus 2 tablespoons sugar*
2 eggs
1¾ cups all-purpose flour

2¾ teaspoons baking powder
1 cup peeled, coarsely
  chopped apple
3 medium bananas, chopped
Vegetable cooking spray

STEPS IN PREPARATION:

1. Cream margarine in a large bowl; gradually add sugar substitute, beating at medium speed of an electric mixer until light and fluffy. Add eggs, and beat until thick and lemon colored.
2. Combine flour and baking powder; add to creamed mixture, mixing well. Fold in apple and banana.
3. Spoon batter into an 8½- x 4½- x 3-inch loafpan coated with cooking spray. Bake at 350° for 65 to 70 minutes or until a wooden pick inserted in center comes out clean.
4. Cool in pan 10 minutes; remove from pan, and cool completely on a wire rack.

Yield: 1 loaf (16 slices)

*See the sugar substitution chart on page 354.

BLUEBERRY LOAF

Exchanges: 1 Starch

Serving Size: 1 (½-inch) slice
Carbohydrate: 14 gm
Protein: 2 gm
Fat: 1 gm

Calories: 74
Fiber: 2 gm
Sodium: 145 mg
Cholesterol: 12 mg

INGREDIENTS:

1 cup all-purpose flour
¾ cup whole wheat flour
2 teaspoons baking powder
½ teaspoon baking soda
½ teaspoon salt
½ cup shreds of wheat bran cereal
⅓ cup granulated brown sugar substitute

¾ cup unsweetened orange juice
1 tablespoon vegetable oil
1 egg
1 cup fresh blueberries
Vegetable cooking spray

STEPS IN PREPARATION:

1. Combine first 7 ingredients in a medium bowl, stirring well. Set aside.
2. Combine orange juice, oil, and egg in a large bowl; beat at medium speed of an electric mixer until well blended. Gradually add flour mixture, stirring just until dry ingredients are moistened. Gently fold in blueberries.
3. Spoon batter into an 8½- x 4½- x 3-inch loafpan coated with cooking spray. Bake at 350° for 50 minutes or until a wooden pick inserted in center comes out clean.
4. Cool in pan 10 minutes; remove from pan, and cool completely on a wire rack.

Yield: 1 loaf (16 slices)

CARROT BREAD

Exchanges: 1 Starch

Serving Size: 1 (½-inch) slice
Carbohydrate: 12 gm
Protein: 2 gm
Fat: 2 gm

Calories: 76
Fiber: 1 gm
Sodium: 87 mg
Cholesterol: 21 mg

INGREDIENTS:

Sugar substitute to equal 2
  cups sugar*
4 eggs
½ cup water
¼ cup vegetable oil
3 cups all-purpose flour

2 teaspoons baking powder
1½ teaspoons baking soda
¼ teaspoon salt
2 teaspoons ground cinnamon
2 cups shredded carrot
Vegetable cooking spray

STEPS IN PREPARATION:

1. Combine sugar substitute and eggs in a large bowl; beat at medium speed of an electric mixer until mixture thickens. Gradually add water and oil; beat well.
2. Combine flour and next 4 ingredients; gradually add to egg mixture, stirring just until dry ingredients are moistened. Fold in carrot.
3. Spoon batter evenly into 2 (9- x 5- x 3-inch) loafpans coated with cooking spray. Bake at 350° for 1 hour or until a wooden pick inserted in center comes out clean.
4. Cool in pans 10 minutes; remove from pans, and cool completely on wire racks.

Yield: 2 loaves (18 slices each)

*See the sugar substitution chart on page 354.

CASSEROLE CHEESE BREAD

Exchanges: 1 Starch, ½ Fat

Serving Size: 1 wedge
Carbohydrate: 15 gm
Protein: 3 gm
Fat: 3 gm

Calories: 96
Fiber: 1 gm
Sodium: 223 mg
Cholesterol: 28 mg

INGREDIENTS:

1 cup all-purpose flour
1 cup whole wheat flour
1 tablespoon baking powder
½ teaspoon salt
Sugar substitute to equal 2
  tablespoons sugar*
1 tablespoon instant minced
  onion
½ teaspoon dried Italian
  seasoning

⅓ cup skim milk
¼ cup reduced-calorie
  margarine, melted
2 eggs, lightly beaten
Vegetable cooking spray
1 tablespoon grated
  Parmesan cheese

STEPS IN PREPARATION:

1. Combine first 7 ingredients in a medium bowl; make a well in center of mixture. Combine milk, margarine, and eggs; add to dry ingredients, stirring just until dry ingredients are moistened.
2. Spoon batter into a round 1½-quart casserole coated with cooking spray. Sprinkle with Parmesan cheese.
3. Bake at 400° for 25 to 30 minutes or until a wooden pick inserted in center comes out clean. Let stand 10 minutes before slicing.

Yield: 1 loaf (18 wedges)

*See the sugar substitution chart on page 354.

MEXICAN CORNBREAD

Exchanges: 1 Starch, 1 Fat

Serving Size: 1 wedge
Carbohydrate: 18 gm
Protein: 5 gm
Fat: 5 gm

Calories: 136
Fiber: 1 gm
Sodium: 327 mg
Cholesterol: 6 mg

INGREDIENTS:

1 cup self-rising cornmeal
1 cup (4 ounces) shredded
   low-fat process American
   cheese
1 cup whole kernel corn
1 cup skim milk
½ cup chopped onion
⅓ cup reduced-calorie
   margarine

2 tablespoons chopped
   jalapeño pepper
½ teaspoon garlic powder
1 (4-ounce) jar diced
   pimiento, drained
Vegetable cooking spray

STEPS IN PREPARATION:

1. Combine first 9 ingredients in a medium bowl, stirring well.
2. Pour batter into a 10½-inch cast-iron skillet coated with cooking
   spray. Bake at 350° for 45 minutes or until golden. Cut into 10
   wedges, and serve warm.

Yield: 10 wedges

CRANBERRY-PECAN BREAD

Exchanges: 1 Starch, ½ Fat

Serving Size: 1 (½-inch) slice	**Calories:** 88
Carbohydrate: 13 gm	**Fiber:** 1 gm
Protein: 2 gm	**Sodium:** 206 mg
Fat: 3 gm	**Cholesterol:** 10 mg

INGREDIENTS:

2 cups all-purpose flour
1 teaspoon baking powder
1 teaspoon salt
½ teaspoon ground cinnamon
½ teaspoon ground nutmeg
1 egg
Liquid sugar substitute to equal 1 cup sugar*
½ cup water
⅓ cup unsweetened orange juice
¼ cup reduced-calorie margarine, melted
3 tablespoons white vinegar
1 teaspoon grated orange rind
1 cup coarsely chopped cranberries
24 small pecans, chopped
Vegetable cooking spray

STEPS IN PREPARATION:

1. Combine first 5 ingredients in a medium bowl.
2. Beat egg; stir in sugar substitute and next 5 ingredients. Add egg mixture to flour mixture, stirring just until dry ingredients are moistened. Fold in cranberries and pecans.
3. Spoon batter into a 9- x 5- x 3-inch loafpan coated with cooking spray. Bake at 350° for 1 hour or until a wooden pick inserted in center comes out clean.
4. Cool in pan 10 minutes. Remove from pan; cool overnight before slicing.

Yield: 1 loaf (18 slices)

*See the sugar substitution chart on page 354.

ORANGE MARMALADE NUT BREAD

Exchanges: 1 Starch

Serving Size: 1 (½-inch) slice
Carbohydrate: 14 gm
Protein: 2 gm
Fat: 2 gm

Calories: 84
Fiber: 1 gm
Sodium: 132 mg
Cholesterol: 11 mg

INGREDIENTS:

2 cups all-purpose flour
1½ teaspoons baking powder
½ teaspoon baking soda
¼ teaspoon salt
½ cup skim milk
Liquid sugar substitute to
   equal ½ cup sugar*
2 tablespoons reduced-calorie
   margarine, melted

1 teaspoon grated orange rind
1 egg, lightly beaten
½ cup low-sugar orange
   marmalade
¼ cup chopped pecans
Vegetable cooking spray

STEPS IN PREPARATION:

1. Combine first 4 ingredients in a medium bowl.
2. Combine milk and next 4 ingredients. Add milk mixture to flour mixture, stirring just until dry ingredients are moistened. Fold in marmalade and nuts.
3. Spoon batter into a 9- x 5- x 3-inch loafpan coated with cooking spray. Bake at 350° for 1 hour and 40 minutes or until a wooden pick inserted in center comes out clean.
4. Remove from pan, and let cool on a wire rack.

Yield: 1 loaf (18 slices)

*See the sugar substitution chart on page 354.

PARKER HOUSE ROLLS

Exchanges: 1 Starch

Serving Size: 1 roll	**Calories:** 75
Carbohydrate: 12 gm	**Fiber:** trace
Protein: 2 gm	**Sodium:** 114 mg
Fat: 2 gm	**Cholesterol:** 23 mg

INGREDIENTS:

3 cups all-purpose flour, divided
1 package dry yeast
Sugar substitute to equal 6 tablespoons sugar*
¾ cup skim milk
⅓ cup reduced-calorie margarine
½ teaspoon salt
2 eggs
Vegetable cooking spray

STEPS IN PREPARATION:

1. Combine 1½ cups flour, yeast, and sugar substitute.
2. Combine skim milk, margarine, and salt in a saucepan; cook over medium heat until margarine melts. Cool to 120° to 130°. Add liquid mixture to flour mixture. Add eggs; beat at low speed of an electric mixer 30 seconds. Increase speed to high; beat 3 minutes. Stir in remaining 1½ cups flour to make a stiff dough.
3. Turn dough out onto a lightly floured surface. Knead until smooth and elastic (about 8 to 10 minutes). Shape into a ball; place in a bowl coated with cooking spray, turning to grease top. Cover and let rise in a warm place (85°), free from drafts, 1 hour or until doubled in bulk. Punch dough down; cover and let rest 10 minutes.
4. Roll dough to ¼-inch thickness; cut with a 2-inch biscuit cutter. Make a crease across each circle, and fold one half over. Gently press edges to seal. Place rolls on baking sheets coated with cooking spray. Cover and let rise in a warm place, free from drafts, until doubled in bulk. Bake at 375° for 15 to 20 minutes or until lightly browned.

Yield: 2 dozen rolls

*See the sugar substitution chart on page 354.

CINNAMON ROLLS

Exchanges: 1½ Starch, ½ Fat

Serving Size: 1 roll **Carbohydrate:** 25 gm **Protein:** 3 gm **Fat:** 2 gm	**Calories:** 128 **Fiber:** 1 gm **Sodium:** 131 mg **Cholesterol:** 16 mg

INGREDIENTS:

4 cups all-purpose flour, divided
1 package dry yeast
Sugar substitute to equal ⅓ cup sugar*
1 cup skim milk
⅓ cup plus 3 tablespoons reduced-calorie margarine, divided

1 teaspoon salt
2 eggs
Vegetable cooking spray
Sugar substitute to equal ½ cup sugar*
2 teaspoons ground cinnamon
¾ cup raisins, divided

STEPS IN PREPARATION:

1. Combine 2 cups flour, yeast, and sugar substitute to equal ⅓ cup sugar.
2. Combine milk, ⅓ cup margarine, and salt in a saucepan; cook over medium heat until margarine melts. Cool to 120° to 130°. Add liquid mixture to flour mixture. Add eggs; beat at low speed of an electric mixer 30 seconds. Increase speed to high; beat 3 minutes. Add remaining 2 cups flour, stirring to make a stiff dough.
3. Turn dough out onto a lightly floured surface. Knead until smooth and elastic (about 8 to 10 minutes). Shape dough into a ball, and place in a bowl coated with cooking spray, turning to grease top. Cover and let rise in a warm place (85°), free from drafts, 1 hour or until doubled in bulk. Punch dough down; divide in half. Cover and let rest 10 minutes.
4. Roll each half of dough to a 12- x 8-inch rectangle. Melt remaining 3 tablespoons margarine; brush half of melted margarine over each rectangle.
5. Combine sugar substitute equal to ½ cup sugar and cinnamon; sprinkle half of cinnamon mixture over each rectangle. Sprinkle each with half of raisins.

6. Roll up rectangles, jellyroll fashion, beginning at long sides; press edges and ends together to seal. Cut each roll into 12 slices. Arrange slices in 9-inch round baking pans coated with cooking spray.
7. Cover and let rise in a warm place, free from drafts, 30 minutes or until doubled in bulk. Bake at 375° for 20 minutes or until lightly browned. Cool slightly; remove from pans, and serve warm.

Yield: 2 dozen rolls

*See the sugar substitution chart on page 354.

Spices aren't just for flavor. USDA (United States Department of Agriculture) scientists found that cinnamon, cloves, and tumeric helped improve blood sugar levels. The spices appeared to help insulin work more effectively in laboratory tests. Although more research is needed to understand just how much of these spices would be needed to help regulate blood sugar, the benefits are just another reason to enjoy their savory touch in your diet.

PEAR-PEPPER RING

Exchanges: 1 Starch

Serving Size: 1 slice	**Calories:** 93
Carbohydrate: 18 gm	**Fiber:** trace
Protein: 3 gm	**Sodium:** 114 mg
Fat: 1 gm	**Cholesterol:** 30 mg

INGREDIENTS:

1 medium-size ripe pear,
   peeled and diced
¼ cup water
1 package dry yeast
Sugar substitute to equal 2
   tablespoons sugar*
1 teaspoon salt

1 teaspoon freshly ground
   pepper
1 egg
3 cups all-purpose flour
Vegetable cooking spray
1 tablespoon skim milk
1 egg yolk

STEPS IN PREPARATION:

1. Combine pear and water in a saucepan; cover and bring to a boil.
   Reduce heat; simmer 10 minutes or until pear is tender. Drain.
2. Place pear in container of an electric blender; cover and process
   until smooth. Transfer pear to a bowl; let cool to 105° to 115°.
3. Sprinkle yeast over pear. Add sugar substitute and next 3 ingredients. Add flour, stirring to make a stiff dough.
4. Turn out onto a floured surface; knead until smooth and elastic.
   Shape into a ball; place in a bowl coated with cooking spray, turning to grease top. Cover and let rise in a warm place (85°), free
   from drafts, 1 hour or until doubled in bulk.
5. Punch dough down. Shape into a ball; place on a baking sheet coated
   with cooking spray. Press dough in center to make a hole 6 inches in
   diameter (dough should resemble a large doughnut). Cover and let
   rise in a warm place, free from drafts, 1 hour or until doubled in bulk.
   Cut ½-inch-deep slashes around top of loaf.
6. Combine milk and egg yolk; brush over loaf. Bake at 375° for 30
   to 35 minutes or until loaf sounds hollow when tapped.

Yield: 1 loaf (18 slices)

*See the sugar substitution chart on page 354.

GARLIC MONKEY BREAD

Exchanges: 1 Starch

Serving Size: 1 slice
Carbohydrate: 16 gm
Protein: 2 gm
Fat: 1 gm

Calories: 80
Fiber: 1 gm
Sodium: 127 mg
Cholesterol: 0 mg

INGREDIENTS:

1 package dry yeast
1 cup warm water (105° to 115°)
3 cups all-purpose flour, divided
1 teaspoon salt
Vegetable cooking spray

1 tablespoon reduced-calorie margarine, melted
1 teaspoon dried parsley flakes
⅛ teaspoon pepper
1 clove garlic, minced

STEPS IN PREPARATION:

1. Dissolve yeast in warm water in a large bowl; let stand 5 minutes.
2. Combine 1½ cups flour and salt; add to yeast mixture, stirring well. Gradually stir in remaining 1½ cups flour to make a stiff dough.
3. Turn dough out onto a lightly floured surface; cover and let rest 10 minutes. Knead until smooth and elastic (about 8 to 10 minutes). Place dough in a bowl coated with cooking spray, turning to grease top. Cover and let rise in a warm place (85°), free from drafts, 1 hour or until doubled in bulk.
4. Combine margarine, parsley, pepper, and garlic, stirring well. Shape dough into 1½-inch balls, and dip each in margarine mixture. Layer balls of dough in a 10-inch ring mold. Cover and let rise in a warm place, free from drafts, 1 hour or until doubled in bulk. Bake at 375° for 25 to 30 minutes or until lightly browned.
5. Cool in pan 5 minutes; invert onto a serving platter, and serve warm.

Yield: 1 loaf (18 slices)

POTATO PANCAKES

Exchanges: 1 Starch, ½ Fat

Serving Size: 2 pancakes
Carbohydrate: 16 gm
Protein: 4 gm
Fat: 3 gm

Calories: 103
Fiber: 1 gm
Sodium: 378 mg
Cholesterol: 47 mg

INGREDIENTS:

3⅓ cups shredded cooked
   potatoes
2 eggs, lightly beaten
¾ cup skim milk
¼ cup chopped onion
2 tablespoons reduced-calorie
   margarine, melted

2 tablespoons all-purpose
   flour
1 teaspoon baking powder
1 teaspoon salt

STEPS IN PREPARATION:

1. Combine potato and eggs; stir well. Add milk and remaining
   ingredients; stir well. Let stand 10 minutes.
2. For each pancake, spoon ¼ cup batter onto a hot nonstick skillet.
   Brown on one side; turn and brown other side.

Yield: 16 pancakes

FRENCH TOAST

Exchanges: 2 Starch, 1 Medium-Fat Meat

Serving Size: 2 slices	**Calories:** 202
Carbohydrate: 26 gm	**Fiber:** 1 gm
Protein: 10 gm	**Sodium:** 578 mg
Fat: 6 gm	**Cholesterol:** 189 mg

INGREDIENTS:

2 eggs
2 teaspoons skim milk
¼ teaspoon salt

4 (1-ounce) slices white bread
Vegetable cooking spray

STEPS IN PREPARATION:

1. Beat eggs. Add milk and salt; beat until frothy.
2. Dip each bread slice into egg mixture, coating well.
3. Place bread slices in a large nonstick skillet coated with cooking spray. Cook 4 to 5 minutes on each side until browned.

Yield: 2 servings

If you want to increase fiber in your diet, switch from white bread and other highly processed wheat products to whole-grain breads and cereals.

FARINA AND FRUIT

Exchanges: 1 Starch

Serving Size: ¼ cup	**Calories:** 62
Carbohydrate: 12 gm	**Fiber:** trace
Protein: 3 gm	**Sodium:** 119 mg
Fat: trace	**Cholesterol:** 1 mg

INGREDIENTS:

1 cup skim milk
⅛ teaspoon salt
2 pitted dates, chopped
2 tablespoons farina,
   uncooked
¼ teaspoon vanilla extract

Sugar substitute to equal 2
   tablespoons sugar*
1 teaspoon reduced-calorie
   margarine
⅛ teaspoon ground cinnamon

STEPS IN PREPARATION:

1. Combine first 3 ingredients in a saucepan; bring to a boil.
   Gradually stir in farina and vanilla. Reduce heat, and simmer, stirring constantly, 2 to 3 minutes or until thickened.
2. Remove from heat; add sugar substitute and margarine, stirring
   until margarine melts.
3. Spoon mixture into serving bowls, and sprinkle evenly with
   cinnamon. Serve warm.

Yield: 4 servings

*See the sugar substitution chart on page 354.

BAKED CHEESE GRITS

Exchanges: 1 Starch, 1 Medium-Fat Meat

Serving Size: ¼ cup
Carbohydrate: 15 gm
Protein: 8 gm
Fat: 5 gm

Calories: 139
Fiber: 0 gm
Sodium: 675 mg
Cholesterol: 68 mg

INGREDIENTS:

1 cup quick-cooking grits, uncooked
⅓ cup skim milk
2 cups (8 ounces) shredded low-fat process American cheese
½ teaspoon hot sauce
½ teaspoon salt
3 eggs, lightly beaten
Vegetable cooking spray

STEPS IN PREPARATION:

1. Cook grits according to package directions, omitting salt.
2. Add milk and next 4 ingredients, stirring well after each addition.
3. Pour into a 1-quart casserole coated with cooking spray. Bake at 325° for 30 to 35 minutes until firm and lightly browned; serve immediately.

Yield: 10 servings

OATMEAL WITH RAISINS AND CINNAMON

Exchanges: 1 Starch

Serving Size: ½ cup	**Calories:** 68
Carbohydrate: 13 gm	**Fiber:** 2 gm
Protein: 2 gm	**Sodium:** 135 mg
Fat: 1 gm	**Cholesterol:** 0 mg

INGREDIENTS:

1½ cups water
2 tablespoons raisins
¼ teaspoon salt

⅔ cup quick-cooking oats, uncooked
1 teaspoon ground cinnamon

STEPS IN PREPARATION:

1. Combine first 3 ingredients in a saucepan; bring to a boil. Stir in oats and cinnamon.
2. Reduce heat, and simmer 1 minute or until water is absorbed.
3. Remove from heat, and serve warm.

Yield: 4 servings

Quick-cooking rolled oats are the same as regular rolled oats except that they are cut and rolled into smaller, thinner pieces. This helps cut the cooking time from 15 minutes for regular oats to 5 minutes for quick-cooking oats. Quick-cooking and regular oats can be used interchangeably in recipes. Instant oats in individual packages aren't interchangeable because they are precooked and dried and often contain sugar, salt, and flavorings.

APPLE-CINNAMON OATMEAL

Exchanges: 1 Starch, 1 Fruit

Serving Size: ½ cup
Carbohydrate: 25 gm
Protein: 3 gm
Fat: 1 gm

Calories: 120
Fiber: 3 gm
Sodium: 347 mg
Cholesterol: 0 mg

INGREDIENTS:

1½ cups water
¼ teaspoon salt
⅔ cup quick-cooking oats, uncooked
2 tablespoons raisins
1 teaspoon ground cinnamon

1 medium apple, peeled and grated
Sugar substitute to taste (optional)

STEPS IN PREPARATION:

1. Bring water and salt to a boil in a saucepan. Stir in oats and next 3 ingredients.
2. Reduce heat. Simmer 1 minute or until water is absorbed.
3. Remove from heat, and serve warm. Sprinkle with sugar substitute, if desired.

Yield: 3 servings

CORNBREAD DRESSING

Exchanges: 2 Starch, ½ Fat

Serving Size: ¾ cup	**Calories:** 174
Carbohydrate: 29 gm	**Fiber:** 2 gm
Protein: 6 gm	**Sodium:** 499 mg
Fat: 3 gm	**Cholesterol:** 17 mg

INGREDIENTS:

3 cups crumbled cornbread
2 cups fat-free chicken broth
1 cup soft breadcrumbs
1 cup finely chopped celery
¾ cup finely chopped onion

½ teaspoon salt
½ teaspoon pepper
½ teaspoon poultry seasoning
2 egg whites
Vegetable cooking spray

STEPS IN PREPARATION:

1. Combine first 9 ingredients in a medium bowl; stir well.
2. Spoon into an 11- x 7- x 2-inch baking dish coated with cooking spray. Bake at 350° for 45 minutes or until lightly browned and set.

Yield: 8 servings

To get soft breadcrumbs, rub fresh bread slices between your hands or crumble fresh bread in a food processor.

SPOONBREAD

Exchanges: 1 Starch, ½ Fat

Serving Size: ½ cup	**Calories:** 110
Carbohydrate: 15 gm	**Fiber:** 1 gm
Protein: 5 gm	**Sodium:** 364 mg
Fat: 4 gm	**Cholesterol:** 48 mg

INGREDIENTS:

1 cup cornmeal
1 teaspoon salt
1 cup water
2 cups warm skim milk

2 eggs, lightly beaten
3 tablespoons reduced-calorie
    margarine, melted
Vegetable cooking spray

STEPS IN PREPARATION:

1. Combine cornmeal and salt in a medium saucepan. Stir in water; gradually add milk, stirring until smooth.
2. Cook over low heat, stirring constantly, until thickened.
3. Spoon a small amount of hot cornmeal mixture into eggs; stir well. Add egg mixture to remaining hot mixture, stirring constantly. Add margarine; stir well.
4. Pour into a 1½-quart baking dish coated with cooking spray. Bake at 375° for 40 to 50 minutes or until lightly browned.

Yield: 8 servings

CHEESE STRAWS

Exchanges: ½ Starch, 1 Fat

Serving Size: 3 straws
Carbohydrate: 7 gm
Protein: 2 gm
Fat: 4 gm

Calories: 72
Fiber: 0 gm
Sodium: 184 mg
Cholesterol: 4 mg

INGREDIENTS:

1 cup all-purpose flour
½ teaspoon baking powder
½ cup reduced-calorie margarine
1 cup (4 ounces) shredded low-fat process American cheese

3 tablespoons cold water
⅛ teaspoon hot sauce

STEPS IN PREPARATION:

1. Combine flour and baking powder in a medium bowl; cut margarine and cheese into flour mixture with a pastry blender until mixture resembles coarse meal. Slowly add water and hot sauce to mixture. Stir with a fork until all ingredients are moistened.
2. Chill mixture 1 hour.
3. Divide dough into 48 equal strips or fill a cookie press and form 48 straws. Place on nonstick cookie sheets. Bake at 375° for 8 to 10 minutes or until lightly browned. Place on wire racks to cool.

Yield: 4 dozen cheese straws

Eggs and Cheese

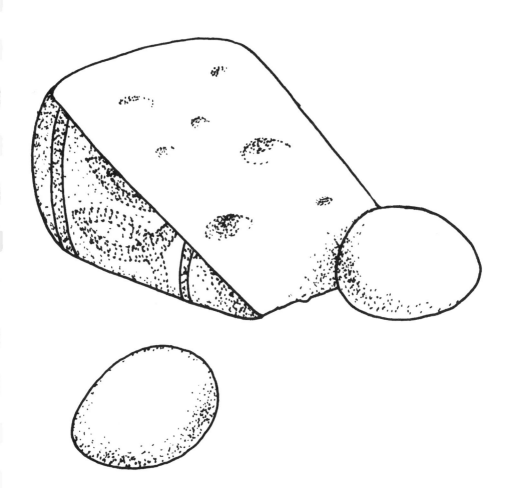

EGG SALAD

Exchanges: 1 Medium-Fat Meat

Serving Size: ⅓ cup
Carbohydrate: 1 gm
Protein: 6 gm
Fat: 6 gm

Calories: 85
Fiber: 0 gm
Sodium: 470 mg
Cholesterol: 187 mg

INGREDIENTS:

6 hard-cooked eggs, diced
½ cup diced celery
2 tablespoons minced green
   pepper
2 tablespoons reduced-calorie
   mayonnaise
1 tablespoon vinegar

1 teaspoon minced onion
1 teaspoon salt
½ teaspoon Worcestershire
   sauce
⅛ teaspoon pepper
Lettuce leaves (optional)

STEPS IN PREPARATION:

1. Combine first 9 ingredients; stir well. Cover and chill.
2. Serve on lettuce leaves, if desired.

Yield: 6 servings

The American Heart Association suggests that you
eat no more than four eggs each week to help keep
dietary cholesterol to a minimum.

DEVILED EGGS

Exchanges: 1 Medium-Fat Meat

Serving Size: 2 egg halves
Carbohydrate: 1 gm
Protein: 6 gm
Fat: 5 gm

Calories: 70
Fiber: 0 gm
Sodium: 221 mg
Cholesterol: 187 mg

INGREDIENTS:

4 hard-cooked eggs, halved
2 teaspoons reduced-calorie
   mayonnaise
1 teaspoon vinegar
½ teaspoon dry mustard

¼ teaspoon salt
Dash of onion powder
Dash of pepper
Paprika

STEPS IN PREPARATION:

1. Remove egg yolks and mash. Set egg white halves aside.
2. Combine yolks, mayonnaise, and next 5 ingredients, stirring well.
3. Pipe yolk mixture into egg white halves. Sprinkle with paprika.
   Cover and chill.

Yield: 4 servings

EGGS BENEDICT

Exchanges: 1 Starch, 2 Medium-Fat Meat

Serving Size: 1 muffin half	**Calories:** 202
Carbohydrate: 19 gm	**Fiber:** 1 gm
Protein: 16 gm	**Sodium:** 657 mg
Fat: 7 gm	**Cholesterol:** 203 mg

INGREDIENTS:

2 whole English muffins
4 (1-ounce) slices lean cooked ham
1 medium tomato, cut into 4 slices
4 eggs, poached and kept warm

¼ cup plus 2 tablespoons plain low-fat yogurt
1 tablespoon lemon juice
1 teaspoon prepared mustard

STEPS IN PREPARATION:

1. Slice muffins in half, and toast.
2. Place 1 ham slice and 1 tomato slice on each muffin half. Broil 4 minutes.
3. Top each muffin half with 1 poached egg.
4. Combine yogurt, lemon juice, and mustard. Spoon 2 tablespoons yogurt mixture over each egg, and serve immediately.

Yield: 4 servings

BAKED EGGS AND MUSHROOMS

Exchanges: 1 Starch, 1 Medium-Fat Meat

Serving Size: ¼ recipe
Carbohydrate: 17 gm
Protein: 8 gm
Fat: 5 gm

Calories: 145
Fiber: 1 gm
Sodium: 375 mg
Cholesterol: 188 mg

INGREDIENTS:

4 eggs, lightly beaten
½ cup skim milk
⅛ teaspoon salt
Dash of pepper
1 cup cooked long-grain rice
  (cooked without salt or fat)

¼ cup canned sliced
  mushrooms, drained
Vegetable cooking spray
Cheese Sauce (page 290)

STEPS IN PREPARATION:

1. Combine first 4 ingredients; stir well. Stir in rice and mushrooms.
2. Pour into an 8-inch square baking dish coated with cooking spray. Bake at 350° for 30 to 35 minutes or until lightly browned and set.
3. To serve, cut into 4 equal portions, and serve with Cheese Sauce.

Yield: 4 servings

Store eggs in the shells for up to five weeks in the refrigerator. Keep them in the carton with large ends up to keep the yolks centered.

EGGS CREOLE

Exchanges: 1 Skim Milk, 1 Fat

Serving Size: 1 cup	**Calories:** 151
Carbohydrate: 15 gm	**Fiber:** 2 gm
Protein: 9 gm	**Sodium:** 416 mg
Fat: 6 gm	**Cholesterol:** 188 mg

INGREDIENTS:

1 tablespoon reduced-calorie margarine
2 teaspoons all-purpose flour
1 cup skim milk
1 cup chopped green pepper
1 cup chopped onion
1 cup canned tomato soup, undiluted

1 teaspoon Worcestershire sauce
6 hard-cooked eggs, coarsely chopped
Vegetable cooking spray
2 tablespoons soft breadcrumbs

STEPS IN PREPARATION:

1. Melt margarine in a small heavy saucepan over low heat; add flour, stirring until smooth. Cook, stirring constantly, 1 minute. Gradually add milk; cook over medium heat, stirring constantly, until mixture is thickened and bubbly. Remove from heat, and set aside.
2. Combine pepper and onion in container of an electric blender or food processor; cover and process until smooth. Transfer mixture to a medium-size nonstick skillet, and cook over low heat 5 minutes.
3. Add soup and Worcestershire sauce to skillet; cook, uncovered, over low heat until thickened.
4. Layer white sauce, eggs, and soup mixture in a 3-quart casserole coated with cooking spray; top with breadcrumbs. Bake at 350° for 20 minutes or until lightly browned and thoroughly heated.

Yield: 6 servings

DEVILED EGG CASSEROLE

Exchanges: ½ Starch, 1½ Medium-Fat Meat

Serving Size: 2 egg halves
Carbohydrate: 9 gm
Protein: 11 gm
Fat: 8 gm

Calories: 152
Fiber: 0 gm
Sodium: 581 mg
Cholesterol: 195 mg

INGREDIENTS:

8 hard-cooked eggs, halved
½ cup reduced-calorie
   mayonnaise
¼ cup chopped mushrooms
¼ teaspoon salt
Vegetable cooking spray
2 tablespoons reduced-calorie
   margarine
2 tablespoons all-purpose
   flour

1½ cups skim milk
½ teaspoon Worcestershire
   sauce
1 cup (4 ounces) shredded
   low-fat process American
   cheese
Paprika

STEPS IN PREPARATION:

1. Remove egg yolks, and mash. Set egg white halves aside.
2. Combine yolks, mayonnaise, mushrooms, and salt.
3. Pipe yolk mixture into egg white halves. Place halves, cut side up, in a 2-quart casserole coated with cooking spray.
4. Melt margarine in a nonstick skillet; add flour, stirring until smooth. Gradually add milk and Worcestershire sauce, stirring constantly. Add cheese, stirring until cheese melts.
5. Pour cheese mixture over eggs; sprinkle with paprika. Bake at 350° for 30 minutes or until bubbly.

Yield: 8 servings

WESTERN-EGG CASSEROLE

Exchanges: 1 Starch, 1 Medium-Fat Meat

Serving Size: ¾ cup
Carbohydrate: 18 gm
Protein: 8 gm
Fat: 5 gm

Calories: 154
Fiber: 2 gm
Sodium: 457 mg
Cholesterol: 144 mg

INGREDIENTS:

1½ cups sliced celery
1 cup chopped green pepper
1 medium onion, sliced
1 tablespoon reduced-calorie margarine, melted
1 tablespoon all-purpose flour
1 teaspoon salt
1 (16-ounce) can low-sodium whole tomatoes, undrained

¼ teaspoon hot sauce
6 hard-cooked eggs, chopped
2 cups cooked long-grain rice (cooked without salt or fat)
Vegetable cooking spray
½ cup (2 ounces) shredded low-fat process American cheese

STEPS IN PREPARATION:

1. Sauté celery, green pepper, and onion in margarine in a 3-quart saucepan until vegetables are tender. Add flour and salt, stirring to blend.
2. Stir in tomatoes and hot sauce; bring to a boil. Reduce heat, and simmer, uncovered, 10 minutes or until mixture is thickened and bubbly, stirring occasionally. Carefully stir in chopped eggs.
3. Spoon rice into a 2-quart casserole coated with cooking spray. Pour egg mixture over rice, and bake, uncovered, at 350° for 25 to 30 minutes or until thoroughly heated. Top with cheese, and bake an additional 5 minutes.

Yield: 8 servings

EGG-RICE CASSEROLE

Exchanges: 1 Starch, 1 Medium-Fat Meat

Serving Size: ⅛ recipe	**Calories:** 135
Carbohydrate: 17 gm	**Fiber:** 1 gm
Protein: 7 gm	**Sodium:** 410 mg
Fat: 4 gm	**Cholesterol:** 164 mg

INGREDIENTS:

7 eggs, lightly beaten
¾ cup skim milk
½ teaspoon celery salt
Dash of pepper
2 cups cooked long-grain rice
   (cooked without salt or fat)

1 (4½-ounce) jar sliced
   mushrooms, drained
Vegetable cooking spray

STEPS IN PREPARATION:

1. Combine first 4 ingredients in a large bowl; stir well. Stir in rice and mushrooms.
2. Pour into an 11- x 7- x 2-inch baking dish coated with cooking spray. Bake at 350° for 30 to 35 minutes or until set. To serve, cut into 8 equal portions.

Yield: 8 servings

Don't wash eggs before storing because washing removes the protective coating that keeps bacteria out of the egg.

HAM OMELET

Exchanges: 2 Medium-Fat Meat

Serving Size: ⅕ omelet
Carbohydrate: 4 gm
Protein: 12 gm
Fat: 9 gm

Calories: 145
Fiber: 1 gm
Sodium: 462 mg
Cholesterol: 305 mg

INGREDIENTS:

8 eggs
½ cup skim milk
1 teaspoon Italian seasoning
½ teaspoon salt
½ teaspoon pepper
½ teaspoon hot sauce

1 tablespoon reduced-calorie margarine
1 medium tomato, chopped
⅓ cup finely chopped lean cooked ham

STEPS IN PREPARATION:

1. Beat first 6 ingredients with a fork until blended (do not overbeat).
2. Melt margarine in a medium nonstick skillet or omelet pan; add egg mixture. As mixture starts to cook, gently lift edges of omelet with a spatula, and tilt pan so uncooked portion flows underneath.
3. When egg mixture is almost set, spoon tomato and ham over half of omelet; continue cooking until eggs are set.
4. Loosen omelet with a spatula, and fold in half; slide onto a serving platter. Divide into 5 equal portions, and serve immediately.

Yield: 5 servings

POTATO-MUSHROOM OMELET

Exchanges: 1 Starch, 1½ Medium-Fat Meat

Serving Size: ¼ omelet	**Calories:** 174
Carbohydrate: 14 gm	**Fiber:** 1 gm
Protein: 14 gm	**Sodium:** 598 mg
Fat: 7 gm	**Cholesterol:** 195 mg

INGREDIENTS:

1 large baking potato, peeled
  and diced
Vegetable cooking spray
½ cup sliced fresh
  mushrooms
½ cup sliced green onions
4 eggs
4 egg whites
½ cup skim milk
½ teaspoon salt
¼ teaspoon pepper
½ cup (2 ounces) shredded
  low-fat process American
  cheese

STEPS IN PREPARATION:

1. Place diced potato in a small saucepan; add boiling water to cover. Cover and cook 10 minutes. Drain well.
2. Coat a 10-inch skillet with cooking spray; place over medium heat until hot. Sauté potato 5 minutes. Add mushrooms and onions, and sauté an additional 5 minutes or until vegetables are tender. Spread potato mixture in bottom of a 9-inch square baking dish coated with cooking spray.
3. Combine eggs and egg whites in a large bowl; beat at medium speed of an electric mixer until frothy. Add milk, salt, and pepper, beating until very light and fluffy.
4. Pour egg mixture over potato mixture, and bake at 350° for 20 to 25 minutes or until lightly browned and puffy. Remove from oven, and top with cheese. Serve immediately.

Yield: 4 servings

COTTAGE CHEESE OMELET

Exchanges: 1 Lean Meat

Serving Size: ½ omelet	**Calories:** 61
Carbohydrate: 1 gm	**Fiber:** trace
Protein: 8 gm	**Sodium:** 667 mg
Fat: 2 gm	**Cholesterol:** 95 mg

INGREDIENTS:

1 egg
2 egg whites
1 tablespoon water
1 teaspoon dried parsley
  flakes
½ teaspoon salt

¼ teaspoon dried marjoram
¼ teaspoon pepper
Vegetable cooking spray
2 tablespoons 1% low-fat
  cottage cheese

STEPS IN PREPARATION:

1. Combine first 7 ingredients in a small bowl, stirring well.
2. Coat a small nonstick skillet with cooking spray; place over medium heat until hot. Pour egg mixture into pan. As mixture starts to cook, gently lift edges of omelet with a spatula, and tilt pan so uncooked portion flows underneath.
3. When egg mixture is almost set, spoon cottage cheese over half of omelet; continue cooking until eggs are set.
4. Loosen omelet with a spatula, and fold in half; slide onto a serving platter, and serve immediately.

Yield: 2 servings

You can refrigerate leftover egg whites and egg yolks. Use raw egg whites within four days and raw egg yolks within one to two days.

CHEESE SOUFFLÉ

Exchanges: 1 Starch, 1 Medium-Fat Meat

Serving Size: ⅓ cup
Carbohydrate: 12 gm
Protein: 10 gm
Fat: 8 gm

Calories: 154
Fiber: 0 gm
Sodium: 631 mg
Cholesterol: 105 mg

INGREDIENTS:

4 (1-ounce) slices white
  bread, cubed
¾ cup skim milk
1 cup (4 ounces) shredded
  low-fat process American
  cheese
2 tablespoons reduced-calorie
  margarine

½ teaspoon salt
½ teaspoon Worcestershire
  sauce
Dash of ground red pepper
3 eggs, separated
Vegetable cooking spray

STEPS IN PREPARATION:

1. Combine bread and milk in a heavy saucepan; bring mixture to a boil. Add cheese and next 4 ingredients.
2. Beat egg yolks; gradually stir about one-fourth of cheese mixture into egg yolks. Stir egg yolk mixture into remaining cheese mixture.
3. Beat egg whites, and fold into cheese mixture.
4. Place mixture in a 1-quart casserole coated with cooking spray; place casserole in a pan of water. Bake at 400° for 35 to 40 minutes or until lightly browned; serve immediately.

Yield: 6 servings

EGGPLANT SOUFFLÉ

Exchanges: 1 Vegetable, 1 Medium-Fat Meat

Serving Size: ½ cup	**Calories:** 88
Carbohydrate: 5 gm	**Fiber:** 1 gm
Protein: 7 gm	**Sodium:** 395 mg
Fat: 5 gm	**Cholesterol:** 78 mg

INGREDIENTS:

3 cups diced eggplant
½ teaspoon salt
1 cup (4 ounces) shredded
   low-fat process American
   cheese
1 cup skim milk

1 tablespoon reduced-calorie
   margarine
⅛ teaspoon hot sauce
Dash of pepper
3 eggs, lightly beaten
Vegetable cooking spray

STEPS IN PREPARATION:

1. Place eggplant in a saucepan with water to cover. Add salt, and cook 8 to 10 minutes or until tender. Drain and cool.
2. Add cheese and next 5 ingredients.
3. Place mixture in a 2-quart casserole coated with cooking spray. Bake at 350° for 30 minutes; serve immediately.

Yield: 8 servings

If you like eggplant, venture beyond the familiar dark purple variety. Several other varieties are also available. Italian eggplant is shaped the same as the standard type but has a delicate skin and fine flesh. White eggplant is usually less bitter than purple eggplant. Slender and straight, Oriental eggplant is often sweeter and smaller than the standard variety.

SPINACH SOUFFLÉ

Exchanges: ½ Medium-Fat Meat, 1 Vegetable

Serving Size: ½ cup	**Calories:** 79
Carbohydrate: 5 gm	**Fiber:** trace
Protein: 6 gm	**Sodium:** 298 mg
Fat: 4 gm	**Cholesterol:** 51 mg

INGREDIENTS:

Vegetable cooking spray
1 tablespoon grated Parmesan cheese
2 tablespoons reduced-calorie margarine
2 tablespoons all-purpose flour
1 cup skim milk
1 teaspoon instant minced onion
¼ teaspoon salt
¼ teaspoon hot sauce
⅛ teaspoon ground nutmeg
2 eggs, separated
1 (10-ounce) package frozen chopped spinach, thawed and well drained
½ cup (2 ounces) shredded low-fat process American cheese
2 egg whites
¾ teaspoon cream of tartar

STEPS IN PREPARATION:

1. Coat bottom of a 2-quart soufflé dish with cooking spray; dust with Parmesan cheese, and set aside.
2. Melt margarine in a 3-quart saucepan over low heat; add flour, stirring until smooth. Cook, stirring constantly, 2 minutes.
3. Gradually add milk and next 4 ingredients; cook over medium heat, stirring constantly, until thickened and bubbly. Remove from heat.
4. Place egg yolks in a small bowl; beat at medium speed of an electric mixer until thick and lemon colored. Gradually stir one-fourth of hot white sauce into egg yolks; stir egg yolk mixture into remaining white sauce. Stir in spinach and shredded cheese. Cook over medium heat 1 minute or until cheese melts.
5. Combine 4 egg whites (at room temperature) and cream of tartar; beat until stiff, but not dry. Gently fold into white sauce mixture.
6. Spoon mixture into prepared dish. Bake at 350° for 50 to 60 minutes or until puffed and browned. Serve immediately.

Yield: 8 servings

CHEESE STRATA

Exchanges: 1 Starch, 2 Medium-Fat Meat

Serving Size: ⅙ recipe	**Calories:** 227
Carbohydrate: 20 gm	**Fiber:** 1 gm
Protein: 16 gm	**Sodium:** 838 mg
Fat: 9 gm	**Cholesterol:** 116 mg

INGREDIENTS:

6 (1-ounce) slices white
  bread, cubed
Vegetable cooking spray
2 cups (8 ounces) shredded
  low-fat process American
  cheese

3 eggs, lightly beaten
2 cups skim milk
¼ teaspoon salt

STEPS IN PREPARATION:

1. Place half of bread cubes in a 1½-quart casserole coated with cooking spray. Layer half of cheese on bread cubes; repeat layers with remaining bread cubes and cheese.
2. Combine eggs, milk, and salt; pour over bread and cheese layers. Cover and chill at least 2 hours.
3. Set casserole in a pan containing ½ inch of hot water. Bake at 325° for 40 to 60 minutes or until a knife inserted in center comes out clean.
4. Cut into 6 equal portions, and serve immediately.

Yield: 6 servings

VEGETARIAN PIZZAS

Exchanges: 2 Starch, 1 Medium-Fat Meat

Serving Size: 1 pizza
Carbohydrate: 32 gm
Protein: 11 gm
Fat: 5 gm

Calories: 203
Fiber: 6 gm
Sodium: 495 mg
Cholesterol: 11 mg

INGREDIENTS:

Vegetable cooking spray
½ cup chopped onion
1 clove garlic, minced
4 cups seeded, chopped tomato
2 tablespoons minced fresh basil
3 tablespoons red wine vinegar
2 teaspoons dried oregano
¼ teaspoon pepper
3 (6-inch) whole wheat pita bread rounds

1 cup (4 ounces) shredded low-fat process American cheese
1 medium-size green pepper, chopped
1 small zucchini, thinly sliced
3 ounces fresh mushrooms, thinly sliced
2 tablespoons grated Parmesan cheese

STEPS IN PREPARATION:

1. Coat a large, heavy skillet with cooking spray; place over medium heat until hot. Add onion and garlic, and sauté until tender.
2. Add tomato and next 4 ingredients to skillet. Bring to a boil; reduce heat, and simmer, uncovered, 20 minutes or until reduced by one-third, stirring occasionally.
3. Separate each pita bread into 2 rounds. Place bread rounds on a baking sheet; bake at 450° for 5 minutes or until lightly browned.
4. Spread ¼ cup tomato mixture over each toasted round. Sprinkle shredded cheese evenly over rounds. Arrange chopped pepper, zucchini, and mushrooms over shredded cheese; sprinkle with Parmesan cheese. Bake at 450° for 10 minutes or until cheese melts.

Yield: 6 servings

ZUCCHINI QUICHE

Exchanges: 1 Medium-Fat Meat, 1 Vegetable

Serving Size: 1 wedge	**Calories:** 107
Carbohydrate: 7 gm	**Fiber:** 1 gm
Protein: 8 gm	**Sodium:** 219 mg
Fat: 5 gm	**Cholesterol:** 94 mg

INGREDIENTS:

1 teaspoon cornstarch
¼ teaspoon dried whole
  oregano
1 cup canned stewed
  tomatoes
1½ cups skim milk
1 tablespoon all-purpose
  flour
4 eggs
2 cups shredded zucchini

½ cup (2 ounces) shredded
  Swiss cheese
½ cup (2 ounces) shredded
  low-fat process American
  cheese
¼ cup chopped onion
2 tablespoons grated
  Parmesan cheese
Vegetable cooking spray

STEPS IN PREPARATION:

1. Combine cornstarch and oregano in a small saucepan. Add tomatoes, stirring well; bring to a boil. Reduce heat, and simmer 2 minutes or until thickened. Set aside, and keep warm.
2. Combine milk, flour, and eggs in a large bowl; beat well using a wire whisk. Add zucchini and next 4 ingredients, stirring well.
3. Pour egg mixture into a 9-inch quiche dish coated with cooking spray. Bake at 350° for 1 hour.
4. Spoon tomato mixture over quiche. Cut into 9 wedges, and serve immediately.

Yield: 9 servings

Fish and Shellfish

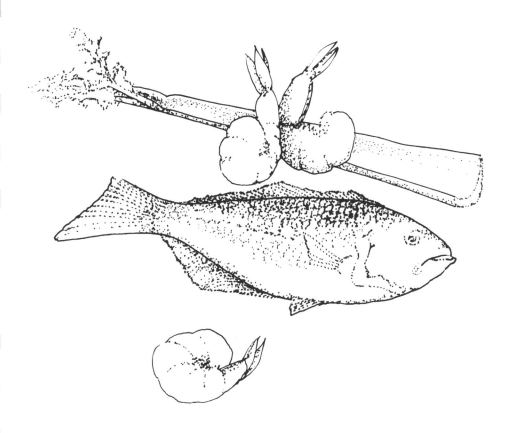

FISH FILLET CASSEROLE

Exchanges: 3 Lean Meat, 1 Vegetable

Serving Size: 3 ounces with sauce	**Calories:** 132
Carbohydrate: 3 gm	**Fiber:** 0 gm
Protein: 19 gm	**Sodium:** 474 mg
Fat: 4 gm	**Cholesterol:** 52 mg

INGREDIENTS:

1½ pounds fish fillets
Vegetable cooking spray
1 (10¾-ounce) can cream of
shrimp soup, undiluted
¼ teaspoon hot sauce

½ cup (2 ounces) shredded
low-fat process American
cheese
½ teaspoon paprika

STEPS IN PREPARATION:

1. Place fillets, skin side down, in a baking dish coated with cooking spray.
2. Combine soup and hot sauce; spoon over fish.
3. Sprinkle with cheese and paprika; bake at 400° for 35 to 45 minutes or until fish flakes easily when tested with a fork.

Yield: 8 servings

Fresh fish is best when cooked the day you buy it. If you need to keep it overnight, rinse the fish with cold water, pat dry, and wrap it in wax paper. Seal the fish in an airtight plastic bag; place the bag in a bowl of ice cubes, and store in the refrigerator.

BROILED FISH FILLETS

Exchanges: 1 Lean Meat

Serving Size: 1 ounce	**Calories:** 43
Carbohydrate: 1 gm	**Fiber:** 0 gm
Protein: 7 gm	**Sodium:** 146 mg
Fat: 1gm	**Cholesterol:** 21 mg

INGREDIENTS:

¼ cup commercial no-oil
  Italian dressing
½ teaspoon Worcestershire
  sauce
¼ teaspoon salt

Dash of pepper
¾ pound fish fillets
1 lime, halved
2 green onions, chopped

STEPS IN PREPARATION:

1. Combine first 4 ingredients; add fillets, and marinate in refrigerator 2 hours.
2. Drain fillets, discarding marinade; place in a broiling pan, and broil 8 to 10 minutes or until fish flakes easily when tested with a fork.
3. Squeeze juice of 1 lime half over fillets; broil 1 minute.
4. Remove fillets from oven, and sprinkle with juice of 1 remaining lime half. Sprinkle with green onions before serving.

Yield: 9 servings

CREOLE FISH FILLETS

Exchanges: 1 Lean Meat, 1 Vegetable

Serving Size: ½ cup	**Calories:** 70
Carbohydrate: 6 gm	**Fiber:** 1 gm
Protein: 9 gm	**Sodium:** 496 mg
Fat: 1 gm	**Cholesterol:** 22 mg

INGREDIENTS:

¾ cup sliced celery
¼ cup chopped onion
1 medium-size green pepper, chopped
1 tablespoon reduced-calorie margarine, melted
1½ cups water
1 (6-ounce) can tomato paste

1 teaspoon salt
¼ teaspoon dried thyme
⅛ teaspoon pepper
Dash of garlic powder
1 bay leaf
2 cups diced cooked fish fillets

STEPS IN PREPARATION:

1. Sauté celery, onion, and green pepper in margarine in a nonstick skillet until vegetables are tender.
2. Add water and next 6 ingredients; simmer 15 minutes, stirring occasionally.
3. Add fillets, and cook until thoroughly heated. Remove and discard bay leaf.
4. Serve fillets over cooked rice (cooked without salt or fat), if desired.

Yield: 8 servings

Note: See the Starch List on page 16 for exchange value of rice.

ORIENTAL BROILED FISH

Exchanges: 1 Lean Meat

Serving Size: 1 ounce	**Calories:** 46
Carbohydrate: 0 gm	**Fiber:** 0 gm
Protein: 7 gm	**Sodium:** 117 mg
Fat: 2 gm	**Cholesterol:** 20 mg

INGREDIENTS:

1 tablespoon vegetable oil
1 tablespoon soy sauce
⅛ teaspoon ground ginger
1 clove garlic, crushed
1 (16-ounce) package frozen unbreaded fish fillets, thawed

2 tablespoons minced green onions

STEPS IN PREPARATION:

1. Combine first 4 ingredients in bottom of a broiling pan. Place fillets in pan, and turn to coat with oil mixture.
2. Cover and marinate in refrigerator at least 1 hour.
3. Broil fillets in marinade 8 to 10 minutes or until fish flakes easily when tested with a fork. Sprinkle with green onions before serving.

Yield: 12 servings

OVEN-FRIED FISH

Exchanges: 2 Lean Meat

Serving Size: 2 ounces	**Calories:** 103
Carbohydrate: 2 gm	**Fiber:** 0 gm
Protein: 16 gm	**Sodium:** 195 mg
Fat: 3 gm	**Cholesterol:** 39 mg

INGREDIENTS:

½ cup crushed corn flakes cereal

½ teaspoon celery salt

⅛ teaspoon onion powder

⅛ teaspoon paprika

Dash of pepper

1 pound catfish or other fish fillets

1 tablespoon plus 1 teaspoon skim milk

Vegetable cooking spray

STEPS IN PREPARATION:

1. Combine first 5 ingredients in a shallow dish.
2. Dip fillets in milk; dredge in cereal mixture.
3. Place fillets in a baking dish coated with cooking spray. Bake at 350° for 25 minutes or until fish is lightly browned and flakes easily when tested with a fork.

Yield: 6 servings

Research shows that fish oils (omega-3 fatty acids) can lower blood pressure and reduce blood clotting. Instead of taking fish oil supplements, add omega-3 fatty acids to your diet by eating salmon, tuna, herring, mackerel, or lake trout twice a week.

BAKED HALIBUT

Exchanges: 3 Lean Meat

Serving Size: 1 steak	**Calories:** 114
Carbohydrate: 1 gm	**Fiber:** trace
Protein: 22 gm	**Sodium:** 220 mg
Fat: 2 gm	**Cholesterol:** 30 mg

INGREDIENTS:

8 (4-ounce) halibut steaks
1 tablespoon Dijon mustard
¼ cup lemon juice
1 tablespoon vinegar
½ teaspoon dried oregano
¼ teaspoon pepper

½ cup water
½ teaspoon chicken-flavored
    bouillon granules
2 green onions, chopped
2 tablespoons grated
    Parmesan cheese

STEPS IN PREPARATION:

1. Rinse steaks thoroughly in cold water; pat dry with paper towels, and place in a shallow baking dish. Brush steaks evenly with mustard.
2. Combine lemon juice, vinegar, oregano, and pepper. Pour over steaks, and marinate in refrigerator 1 to 2 hours.
3. Combine water and bouillon granules in a small saucepan. Cook over medium heat, stirring constantly, until granules dissolve.
4. Pour broth around steaks in marinade in dish. Top steaks with green onions and cheese. Bake at 375° for 25 minutes or until fish flakes easily when tested with a fork.

Yield: 8 servings

HALIBUT FLORENTINE

Exchanges: 2 Lean Meat, 1 Vegetable

Serving Size: ⅛ recipe
Carbohydrate: 5 gm
Protein: 14 gm
Fat: 3 gm

Calories: 105
Fiber: trace
Sodium: 122 mg
Cholesterol: 58 mg

INGREDIENTS:

- 1 (10-ounce) package frozen chopped spinach
- 2 tablespoons lemon juice
- 4 (4-ounce) halibut fillets
- 1 tablespoon reduced-calorie margarine
- 2 tablespoons all-purpose flour
- 1 cup skim milk
- 1 egg yolk, lightly beaten
- ¼ cup (1 ounce) shredded reduced-fat Swiss cheese
- 1 tablespoon grated Parmesan cheese

STEPS IN PREPARATION:

1. Cook spinach according to package directions, omitting salt. Drain well, and place in an 11- x 7- x 2-inch baking dish; sprinkle with lemon juice.
2. Rinse fillets thoroughly in cold water; pat dry with paper towels, and arrange over spinach.
3. Melt margarine in a small saucepan over low heat; add flour, stirring until smooth. Cook, stirring constantly, 1 minute. Gradually add milk; cook over medium heat, stirring constantly, until mixture is thickened and bubbly. Remove from heat, and stir in egg yolk. Add Swiss cheese, and cook over low heat until cheese melts, stirring frequently.
4. Spoon sauce over fillets, and sprinkle with Parmesan cheese. Bake at 350° for 20 minutes or until fish flakes easily when tested with a fork.

Yield: 8 servings

STUFFED FLOUNDER

Exchanges: 1½ Lean Meat, 1 Vegetable

Serving Size: 1 fillet
Carbohydrate: 5 gm
Protein: 13 gm
Fat: 2 gm

Calories: 100
Fiber: 1 gm
Sodium: 120 mg
Cholesterol: 36 mg

INGREDIENTS:

4 (3-ounce) flounder fillets
Vegetable cooking spray
½ cup finely chopped onion
1 clove garlic, minced
¼ cup finely chopped celery
¼ cup finely chopped carrot
¼ cup minced sweet red
  pepper
2 tablespoons chopped fresh
  parsley, divided

⅛ teaspoon ground thyme
1 tablespoon grated
  Parmesan cheese
1 tablespoon reduced-calorie
  mayonnaise
½ teaspoon Dijon mustard
1 tablespoon lemon juice

STEPS IN PREPARATION:

1. Rinse fillets thoroughly in cold water; pat dry with paper towels. Set aside.
2. Coat a medium skillet with cooking spray; place over medium heat until hot. Add onion and garlic; sauté until tender. Add celery, carrot, and pepper; cover and cook over medium-low heat 5 minutes or until vegetables are tender, stirring occasionally. Add 1 tablespoon parsley and thyme.
3. Spoon mixture evenly into centers of fillets; roll up lengthwise, and secure with wooden picks. Place rolls, seam side down, in a shallow baking dish coated with cooking spray.
4. Combine cheese, mayonnaise, and mustard; spread mixture evenly over rolls, and sprinkle with lemon juice. Bake at 400° for 20 minutes or until fish is lightly browned and flakes easily when tested with a fork. Sprinkle with remaining 1 tablespoon parsley. Serve immediately.

Yield: 4 servings

CURRIED FLOUNDER

Exchanges: 2 Lean Meat

Serving Size: 1 fillet
Carbohydrate: 2 gm
Protein: 15 gm
Fat: 2 gm

Calories: 87
Fiber: trace
Sodium: 82 mg
Cholesterol: 42 mg

INGREDIENTS:

8 (3-ounce) flounder fillets
2 green onions, minced
2 small cloves garlic, minced
⅛ teaspoon curry powder
⅛ teaspoon red pepper

2 tablespoons all-purpose
   flour
1 tablespoon reduced-calorie
   margarine

STEPS IN PREPARATION:

1. Rinse fillets thoroughly in cold water; pat dry with paper towels, and place in a shallow baking dish.
2. Combine green onions and next 3 ingredients; rub over fillets. Cover and chill 1 hour.
3. Remove fillets from baking dish, and coat with flour.
4. Melt margarine in baking dish in a 350° oven; add fillets, turning once. Bake for 8 to 10 minutes or until fish flakes easily when tested with a fork.

Yield: 8 servings

Cooking time is critical with fish because the flesh is so delicate. Perfectly cooked fish will be moist and tender; overcooked fish will be dry and tough. When fish is cooked to perfection, the translucent flesh turns opaque (or solid) in appearance, and it flakes easily with a fork.

BAKED SALMON

Exchanges: 2 Lean Meat

Serving Size: 1 steak	**Calories:** 103
Carbohydrate: 1 gm	**Fiber:** trace
Protein: 15 gm	**Sodium:** 44 mg
Fat: 4 gm	**Cholesterol:** 46 mg

INGREDIENTS:

4 (2½-ounce) salmon steaks
Vegetable cooking spray
2 tablespoons lemon juice
½ teaspoon dried dillweed

½ teaspoon dried parsley
   flakes
½ teaspoon pepper

STEPS IN PREPARATION:

1. Rinse steaks thoroughly in cold water; pat dry with paper towels.
2. Place steaks in a shallow pan coated with cooking spray; brush with lemon juice. Sprinkle evenly with dillweed, parsley, and pepper.
3. Bake at 350° for 25 to 35 minutes or until fish flakes easily when tested with a fork.

Yield: 4 servings

SALMON CROQUETTES

Exchanges: 1 Starch, 3 Lean Meat

Serving Size: 1 croquette	**Calories:** 192
Carbohydrate: 12 gm	**Fiber:** 0 gm
Protein: 21 gm	**Sodium:** 274 mg
Fat: 6 gm	**Cholesterol:** 51 mg

INGREDIENTS:

1 (16-ounce) can no-salt-added salmon
⅔ cup skim milk
2 teaspoons reduced-calorie margarine
2 tablespoons minced onion
¼ cup all-purpose flour

¾ teaspoon hot sauce
¼ teaspoon salt
Dash of pepper
1 tablespoon lemon juice
1 cup crushed corn flakes cereal, divided
5 lemon wedges (optional)

STEPS IN PREPARATION:

1. Drain salmon, reserving liquid; add milk to salmon liquid.
2. Melt margarine in a nonstick skillet; add onion, and sauté until tender. Add flour and next 3 ingredients to onion mixture; stir well. Add milk mixture, and cook over low heat, stirring constantly, until thickened.
3. Flake salmon; add salmon and lemon juice to sauce. Stir in ½ cup cereal.
4. Cover and chill 1 hour.
5. Divide mixture into ½-cup portions, and shape into cones; roll cones in remaining ½ cup cereal, coating well.
6. Place on a nonstick baking sheet, and bake at 400° for 20 to 25 minutes or until lightly browned. Garnish with lemon wedges, if desired.

Yield: 5 servings

LEMON-BAKED SOLE

Exchanges: 2 Lean Meat

Serving Size: 1 fillet
Carbohydrate: 3 gm
Protein: 16 gm
Fat: 2 gm

Calories: 98
Fiber: trace
Sodium: 91 mg
Cholesterol: 43 mg

INGREDIENTS:

4 (4-ounce) sole fillets
2 teaspoons reduced-calorie
  margarine, melted
2 teaspoons lemon juice
2 tablespoons all-purpose
  flour

2 teaspoons chopped fresh
  parsley
⅛ teaspoon pepper
⅛ teaspoon paprika
Lemon wedges (optional)
Fresh parsley sprigs (optional)

STEPS IN PREPARATION:

1. Rinse fillets thoroughly in cold water; pat dry with paper towels, and set aside.
2. Combine margarine and lemon juice in a small bowl. Combine flour, chopped parsley, and pepper in a shallow dish. Dip fillets in margarine mixture, and dredge in flour mixture.
3. Transfer fillets to a nonstick baking sheet, and drizzle remaining margarine mixture over fillets. Sprinkle with paprika.
4. Bake at 375° for 15 to 20 minutes or until fish is golden and flakes easily when tested with a fork. If desired, garnish with lemon wedges and parsley sprigs.

Yield: 4 servings

VEGETABLE-TOPPED SNAPPER

Exchanges: 3 Lean Meat, 1 Vegetable

Serving Size: 1 fillet	**Calories:** 162
Carbohydrate: 6 gm	**Fiber:** 1 gm
Protein: 23 gm	**Sodium:** 403 mg
Fat: 5 gm	**Cholesterol:** 61 mg

INGREDIENTS:

6 (4-ounce) snapper fillets
½ teaspoon dried tarragon
¼ teaspoon salt
¼ teaspoon pepper
Vegetable cooking spray
1 medium onion, chopped
¼ pound fresh mushrooms, sliced

3 tablespoons reduced-calorie margarine, melted
1 medium tomato, seeded and chopped
¼ cup reduced-calorie ketchup
2 tablespoons grated Parmesan cheese

STEPS IN PREPARATION:

1. Rinse fillets thoroughly in cold water; pat dry with paper towels.
2. Sprinkle fillets with tarragon, salt, and pepper, and place in a 13- x 9- x 2-inch baking dish coated with cooking spray. Bake, uncovered, at 500° for 10 to 12 minutes or until fish flakes easily when tested with a fork.
3. Sauté onion and mushrooms in margarine in a large skillet until vegetables are tender. Remove from heat, and stir in tomato and ketchup.
4. Remove fillets from oven; drain. Spoon onion mixture evenly over fillets, and sprinkle with cheese. Broil 3 inches from heat until cheese melts. Serve immediately.

Yield: 6 servings

TUNA CREOLE

Exchanges: 2 Lean Meat, 2 Vegetable

Serving Size: 1 cup	**Calories:** 136
Carbohydrate: 9 gm	**Fiber:** 2 gm
Protein: 18 gm	**Sodium:** 679 mg
Fat: 3 gm	**Cholesterol:** 10 mg

INGREDIENTS:

1 cup chopped onion
2 tablespoons chopped green pepper
2 tablespoons reduced-calorie margarine, melted
2 tablespoons all-purpose flour
1 (14½-ounce) can tomatoes
¼ cup sliced stuffed olives
½ teaspoon dried oregano
½ teaspoon salt
⅛ teaspoon pepper
⅛ teaspoon ground allspice
2 (6½-ounce) cans tuna in water

STEPS IN PREPARATION:

1. Sauté onion and green pepper in margarine in a nonstick skillet until vegetables are tender.
2. Add flour; stirring well. Add tomatoes and next 5 ingredients; cook, stirring constantly, until thickened.
3. Drain and flake tuna; stir into tomato mixture.
4. Serve over cooked rice or noodles (cooked without salt or fat), if desired.

Yield: 6 servings

Note: See the Starch List on page 16 for exchange values of rice and noodles.

TUNA SALAD

Exchanges: 2 Lean Meat

Serving Size: ½ cup
Carbohydrate: 2 gm
Protein: 15 gm
Fat: 2 gm

Calories: 95
Fiber: 0 gm
Sodium: 283 mg
Cholesterol: 101 mg

INGREDIENTS:

1 (6½-ounce) can tuna in
   water, drained and flaked
2 hard-cooked eggs, chopped
¼ cup chopped celery

2 tablespoons nonfat
   mayonnaise
Lettuce leaves (optional)

STEPS IN PREPARATION:

1. Combine first 4 ingredients in a small bowl. Cover and chill.
2. Serve on lettuce leaves, if desired.

Yield: 4 servings

Canned tuna is available in the following forms:
tuna packed in oil or spring water, chunk or solid
pack, and light tuna or albacore tuna. Tuna packed
in water contains 36 calories per ounce versus 82
calories for the same amount of tuna packed in oil.

CHOPSTICK TUNA

Exchanges: 1 Starch, 1 Lean Meat

Serving Size: 1 cup	**Calories:** 131
Carbohydrate: 16 gm	**Fiber:** 3 gm
Protein: 10 gm	**Sodium:** 453 mg
Fat: 3 gm	**Cholesterol:** 4 mg

INGREDIENTS:

1 (6½-ounce) can tuna in water, drained and flaked
½ cup skim milk
¼ cup water
½ (10¾-ounce) can cream of mushroom soup, undiluted
1 (10-ounce) package frozen English peas
1 (8-ounce) can sliced water chestnuts, drained
1½ ounces chow mein noodles, divided
1 medium tomato, diced
½ cup chopped celery
¼ cup sliced green onions
2 tablespoons reduced-sodium soy sauce
Vegetable cooking spray

STEPS IN PREPARATION:

1. Place tuna in a medium bowl. Combine milk, water, and soup; add to tuna, stirring well. Add peas, water chestnuts, half of noodles, and next 4 ingredients; toss lightly to mix.
2. Spoon mixture into a 1½-quart casserole coated with cooking spray; top with remaining noodles. Bake at 375° for 25 to 30 minutes or until thoroughly heated.

Yield: 8 servings

Microwave Note: Microwave at HIGH for 5 minutes; rotate dish a half turn, and microwave at MEDIUM (50% power) for 3 to 5 minutes or until thoroughly heated.

STIR-FRIED TUNA

Exchanges: 1 Starch, 2 Lean Meat

Serving Size: ¾ cup
Carbohydrate: 12 gm
Protein: 18 gm
Fat: trace

Calories: 126
Fiber: 2 gm
Sodium: 522 mg
Cholesterol: 10 mg

INGREDIENTS:

Vegetable cooking spray
1 medium-size sweet red or green pepper, coarsely chopped
8 green onions, cut into ½-inch pieces
1 clove garlic, minced
1 cup diagonally sliced celery
5 ounces fresh snow pea pods
2 ounces fresh mushrooms, sliced

1 (8-ounce) can sliced water chestnuts, drained
1 tablespoon cornstarch
3 tablespoons reduced-sodium soy sauce
3 tablespoons water
1 tablespoon vinegar
¼ teaspoon ground ginger
2 (6½-ounce) cans tuna in water, drained and flaked

STEPS IN PREPARATION:

1. Coat a wok or large heavy skillet with cooking spray; heat at medium-high (375°) for 2 minutes. Add pepper, green onions, and garlic; stir-fry 15 seconds. Add celery and next 3 ingredients; stir-fry 1 minute or until vegetables are crisp-tender.
2. Combine cornstarch and next 4 ingredients, stirring until cornstarch dissolves; add to wok. Cook over medium-high heat until sauce is slightly thickened, stirring frequently. Add tuna, stirring to coat well.
3. Serve over cooked rice (cooked without salt or fat), if desired.

Yield: 6 servings

Note: See the Starch List on page 16 for exchange value of rice.

TUNA PILAF

Exchanges: 1 Starch, 1 Lean Meat, 1 Vegetable

Serving Size: ½ cup	**Calories:** 275
Carbohydrate: 18 gm	**Fiber:** 2 gm
Protein: 14 gm	**Sodium:** 454 mg
Fat: 1 gm	**Cholesterol:** 13 mg

INGREDIENTS:

2 green onions, chopped
1 teaspoon reduced-calorie margarine, melted
2½ cups water
1 cup long-grain rice, uncooked
1 (10-ounce) package frozen mixed Oriental vegetables, thawed
1 (10-ounce) can tuna in water, drained and broken into chunks
1 tablespoon reduced-sodium soy sauce

STEPS IN PREPARATION:

1. Sauté onions in margarine in a large saucepan until onions are tender.
2. Add water; bring to a boil. Stir in rice; cover, reduce heat, and simmer 20 to 25 minutes or until rice is tender and liquid is absorbed.
3. Add mixed vegetables. Cook over low heat 5 minutes or until vegetables are tender.
4. Add tuna and soy sauce; stir. Serve warm.

Yield: 8 servings

SHRIMP SALAD

Exchanges: 2 Lean Meat, 1 Vegetable

Serving Size: ⅓ cup	**Calories:** 96
Carbohydrate: 4 gm	**Fiber:** 0 gm
Protein: 17 gm	**Sodium:** 393 mg
Fat: 1 gm	**Cholesterol:** 161 mg

INGREDIENTS:

3 cups water
1 pound unpeeled medium-
   size fresh shrimp
¼ cup nonfat mayonnaise
¾ teaspoon diced pimiento
¾ teaspoon lemon juice

½ teaspoon prepared
   mustard
⅛ teaspoon ground white
   pepper
⅛ teaspoon chopped parsley
⅓ cup finely chopped celery

STEPS IN PREPARATION:

1. Bring 3 cups water to a boil in a medium saucepan. Add shrimp;
   cook 5 minutes or until shrimp turns pink. Drain well; cool. Peel
   and devein shrimp; chop.
2. Combine mayonnaise and next 5 ingredients; stir well.
3. Add shrimp and celery to mayonnaise mixture. Cover and chill.

Yield: 4 servings

The key to lowering blood cholesterol is to cut
down on high-cholesterol foods and foods that are
high in saturated fat.

Although shrimp is higher in cholesterol than
some other types of shellfish, it is very low in saturated fat. A 3-ounce portion of shrimp contains 166
milligrams of cholesterol, so you can include
shrimp in your diet and still stay below the
American Heart Association's recommendation of
no more than 300 milligrams of cholesterol per day.

SHRIMP-MACARONI SALAD

Exchanges: ½ Starch, 1 Lean Meat

Serving Size: ¾ cup	**Calories:** 100
Carbohydrate: 11 gm	**Fiber:** 1 gm
Protein: 6 gm	**Sodium:** 212 mg
Fat: 4 gm	**Cholesterol:** 42 mg

INGREDIENTS:

- ¾ cup uncooked shell macaroni
- 3 cups water
- ¾ pound medium-size fresh shrimp, peeled and deveined
- 1 cup chopped cauliflower
- 1 cup sliced celery
- ½ cup commercial low-calorie French dressing
- ¼ cup chopped fresh parsley
- ¼ cup chopped sweet pickle
- ¼ cup reduced-calorie mayonnaise
- 1 tablespoon lemon juice
- 1 teaspoon grated onion
- ½ teaspoon celery seeds
- ¼ teaspoon pepper

STEPS IN PREPARATION:

1. Cook macaroni according to package directions, omitting salt and fat. Drain and set aside.
2. Bring 3 cups water to a boil in a medium saucepan. Add shrimp; cook 3 to 5 minutes or until shrimp turns pink. Drain well.
3. Combine macaroni, shrimp, cauliflower, and remaining ingredients; toss gently to combine. Cover and chill at least 8 hours.

Yield: 12 servings

SHRIMP SCAMPI

Exchanges: 2 Lean Meat

Serving Size: ¼ recipe	**Calories:** 93
Carbohydrate: 5 gm	**Fiber:** 0 gm
Protein: 15 gm	**Sodium:** 693 mg
Fat: 1 gm	**Cholesterol:** 125 mg

INGREDIENTS:

3 cups water
¾ pound medium-size fresh shrimp, peeled and deveined
1½ cups fat-free chicken broth
½ cup dry butter substitute
1½ tablespoons lemon juice
½ teaspoon salt
½ teaspoon garlic powder
½ teaspoon dried parsley flakes
¼ teaspoon dried oregano leaves
¼ teaspoon dried basil
⅛ teaspoon ground red pepper
1 tablespoon cornstarch

STEPS IN PREPARATION:

1. Bring 3 cups water to a boil in a medium saucepan. Add shrimp; cook 3 minutes. Drain well, and set aside.
2. Combine broth and next 8 ingredients in a medium saucepan. Bring to a boil, and add shrimp. Add cornstarch; cook, stirring constantly, until thickened.
3. Serve over cooked rice (cooked without salt or fat), if desired.

Yield: 4 servings

Note: See the Starch List on page 16 for exchange value of rice.

SHRIMP AND CHICKEN CREOLE

Exchanges: 3 Lean Meat, 2 Vegetable

Serving Size: 1 cup	**Calories:** 140
Carbohydrate: 9 gm	**Fiber:** 2 gm
Protein: 20 gm	**Sodium:** 326 mg
Fat: 3 gm	**Cholesterol:** 122 mg

INGREDIENTS:

1 cup chopped green pepper
¾ cup chopped onion
1 teaspoon vegetable oil
2 cups peeled, diced tomato
½ teaspoon salt
½ teaspoon garlic powder
½ teaspoon chili powder
¼ teaspoon ground red pepper

⅛ teaspoon black pepper
¾ pound small fresh shrimp, peeled and deveined
1 cup chopped cooked chicken (skinned before cooking and cooked without salt)

STEPS IN PREPARATION:

1. Sauté green pepper and onion in oil in a skillet until vegetables are tender.
2. Stir in tomato and next 5 ingredients. Bring to a boil. Reduce heat, and simmer, uncovered, 20 to 30 minutes or until thickened.
3. Stir in shrimp and chicken (mixture will thin when shrimp is added). Return to a boil; reduce heat, and cook 1 to 2 minutes or until shrimp turns pink.
4. Serve over cooked rice (cooked without salt or fat), if desired.

Yield: 6 servings

Note: See the Starch List on page 16 for exchange value of rice.

CURRY-SHRIMP CREOLE

Exchanges: 1 Lean Meat, 1½ Vegetable

Serving Size: ½ cup	**Calories:** 80
Carbohydrate: 8 gm	**Fiber:** 1 gm
Protein: 8 gm	**Sodium:** 393 mg
Fat: 2 gm	**Cholesterol:** 61 mg

INGREDIENTS:

2 medium onions, chopped
1 medium-size green pepper, cut into 1-inch pieces
1 stalk celery, sliced
1 clove garlic, minced
1 tablespoon vegetable oil
1 (16-ounce) can whole tomatoes, undrained and chopped
¼ cup minced fresh parsley
¼ cup reduced-calorie ketchup
1 teaspoon lemon juice
½ teaspoon salt
½ teaspoon hot sauce
¼ teaspoon curry powder
¼ teaspoon dried thyme
¾ pound medium-size fresh shrimp, peeled and deveined

STEPS IN PREPARATION:

1. Sauté first 4 ingredients in oil in a large skillet until vegetables are crisp-tender.
2. Stir in tomato and next 7 ingredients. Cover and bring to a boil. Reduce heat, and simmer 30 minutes.
3. Add shrimp. Cover and simmer 5 minutes or until shrimp turns pink.
4. Serve over cooked rice (cooked without salt or fat), if desired.

Yield: 8 servings

Note: See the Starch List on page 16 for exchange value of rice.

SHRIMP STIR-FRY

Exchanges: 2 Lean Meat, 1 Vegetable

Serving Size: ¾ cup
Carbohydrate: 7 gm
Protein: 14 gm
Fat: 3 gm

Calories: 112
Fiber: 2 gm
Sodium: 362 mg
Cholesterol: 107 mg

INGREDIENTS:

1 tablespoon vegetable oil
1 medium onion, thinly sliced
½ cup thinly sliced celery
1 pound medium-size fresh
   shrimp, peeled and
   deveined
6 ounces fresh mushrooms,
   sliced
½ teaspoon minced garlic

1 cup shredded fresh spinach
4 ounces frozen English peas,
   thawed
1 teaspoon cornstarch
¼ cup water
2 tablespoons reduced-
   sodium soy sauce

STEPS IN PREPARATION:

1. Coat a wok or large heavy skillet with oil. Heat at medium-high (375°) 2 minutes.
2. Add onion and celery to wok; stir-fry 3 minutes. Add shrimp, mushrooms, and garlic; stir-fry 1 minute or until shrimp turns pink. Add spinach and English peas; stir-fry 30 seconds.
3. Combine cornstarch, water, and soy sauce, stirring until cornstarch dissolves; add to shrimp mixture in wok. Cook, stirring constantly, over medium-high heat until mixture thickens.
4. Serve over hot cooked brown rice (cooked without salt or fat), if desired.

Yield: 6 servings

Note: See the Starch List on page 16 for exchange value of brown rice.

SEAFOOD NEWBURG

Exchanges: ½ Starch, 3 Lean Meat

Serving Size: ¾ cup	**Calories:** 155
Carbohydrate: 8 gm	**Fiber:** 0 gm
Protein: 26 gm	**Sodium:** 565 mg
Fat: 2 gm	**Cholesterol:** 126 mg

INGREDIENTS:

3 cups fat-free chicken broth
1 pound medium-size fresh
 shrimp, peeled and deveined
¾ pound scallops
½ cup dry butter substitute
½ teaspoon garlic powder
½ teaspoon dried parsley
 flakes

¼ teaspoon salt
¼ teaspoon ground white
 pepper
¼ teaspoon dried thyme
¼ teaspoon dried sage
3 tablespoons cornstarch
3 tablespoons water
2 tablespoons lemon juice

STEPS IN PREPARATION:

1. Bring broth to a boil in a medium saucepan. Add shrimp and scallops; cook 3 to 5 minutes or until shrimp turns pink. Remove seafood from broth; set seafood aside.
2. Add butter substitute and next 6 ingredients to broth; bring to a boil.
3. Combine cornstarch and water; add to chicken broth mixture. Reduce heat, and simmer 5 minutes. Add lemon juice to broth mixture; add shrimp and scallops, and stir.
4. Serve over cooked rice (cooked without salt or fat), if desired.

Yield: 6 servings

Note: See the Starch List on page 16 for exchange value of rice.

Meats

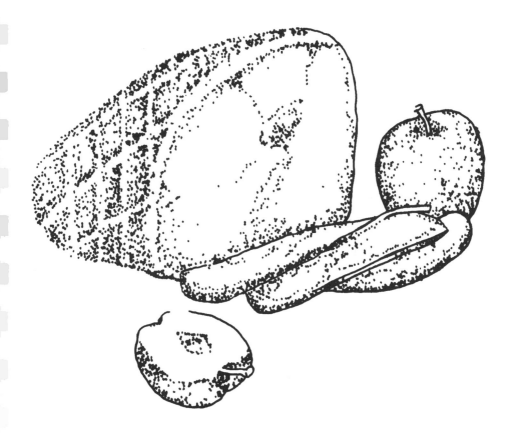

BEEFY CHILI

Exchanges: 1 Starch, 1 Medium-Fat Meat

Serving Size: ½ cup	**Calories:** 118
Carbohydrate: 11 gm	**Fiber:** 4 gm
Protein: 9 gm	**Sodium:** 295 mg
Fat: 4 gm	**Cholesterol:** 16 mg

INGREDIENTS:

1 pound lean ground beef
½ cup chopped onion
1 tablespoon chili powder
1 teaspoon salt
1 (16-ounce) can crushed
   tomatoes, undrained

1 (15-ounce) can kidney
   beans, undrained
3 cups water

STEPS IN PREPARATION:

1. Combine first 4 ingredients in a nonstick skillet. Cook over medium heat until meat is browned, stirring until meat crumbles. Drain and pat dry with paper towels.
2. Combine tomato and beans in a saucepan. Add water.
3. Add meat mixture to saucepan. Bring to a boil; reduce heat, and simmer, uncovered, 1 hour.

Yield: 16 servings

GROUND BEEF PIE

Exchanges: 1 Starch, 2 Medium-Fat Meat

Serving Size: ⅛ recipe
Carbohydrate: 18 gm
Protein: 17 gm
Fat: 8 gm

Calories: 216
Fiber: 6 gm
Sodium: 783 mg
Cholesterol: 33 mg

INGREDIENTS:

1 pound lean ground beef
1 small onion, finely chopped
1 teaspoon salt
½ teaspoon chili powder
⅛ teaspoon pepper
Vegetable cooking spray

1 cup tomato juice
1 (16-ounce) can green beans,
   drained
2½ cups mashed potatoes
   (cooked without salt or fat)
¼ teaspoon paprika

STEPS IN PREPARATION:

1. Combine first 5 ingredients in a nonstick skillet. Cook over medium heat until meat is browned, stirring until meat crumbles. Drain and pat dry with paper towels.
2. Place meat mixture in a 2-quart casserole coated with cooking spray. Pour tomato juice over meat mixture.
3. Arrange beans over meat mixture.
4. Spoon mashed potatoes over beans. Sprinkle with paprika. Bake at 350° for 35 to 40 minutes or until golden.

Yield: 8 servings

ENCHILADA PIE

Exchanges: 2 Medium-Fat Meat, 1 Vegetable

Serving Size: ½ cup	**Calories:** 180
Carbohydrate: 8 gm	**Fiber:** 1 gm
Protein: 14 gm	**Sodium:** 356 mg
Fat: 10 gm	**Cholesterol:** 38 mg

INGREDIENTS:

1 pound ground chuck
½ cup chopped onion
1 (4-ounce) can tomato sauce
1 teaspoon chili powder
½ teaspoon ground cumin
¼ teaspoon salt
¼ teaspoon pepper

4 (6-inch) corn tortillas
¾ cup (3 ounces) shredded
  low-fat process American
  cheese
Vegetable cooking spray
½ cup water

STEPS IN PREPARATION:

1. Cook ground chuck and onion in a large nonstick skillet over medium heat until browned, stirring until meat crumbles. Drain and pat dry with paper towels.
2. Return meat to skillet; stir in tomato sauce and next 4 ingredients. Cook over medium heat, stirring constantly, until thoroughly heated.
3. Layer tortillas, meat sauce, and cheese in a 2-quart casserole coated with cooking spray; pour water over top. Cover and bake at 400° for 20 minutes. Serve warm.

Yield: 8 servings

SAVORY HASH

Exchanges: 2 Medium-Fat Meat, 1 Vegetable

Serving Size: ½ cup
Carbohydrate: 13 gm
Protein: 16 gm
Fat: 11 gm

Calories: 214
Fiber: 2 gm
Sodium: 477 mg
Cholesterol: 43 mg

INGREDIENTS:

1 pound lean ground beef
½ cup finely chopped celery
½ cup finely chopped onion
¼ cup finely chopped green pepper
2 cups chopped tomato

½ cup cooked long-grain rice (cooked without salt or fat)
1 teaspoon chili powder
1 teaspoon salt
¼ teaspoon pepper

STEPS IN PREPARATION:

1. Cook first 4 ingredients in a nonstick skillet over medium heat until meat is browned, stirring until meat crumbles. Drain and pat dry with paper towels.
2. Return meat mixture to skillet; add tomato and remaining ingredients. Cover and cook over low heat 45 minutes, adding water occasionally to keep meat from sticking to skillet.

Yield: 6 servings

For maximum reduction of fat, use ultra-lean ground beef. Consider this difference: a 3-ounce cooked portion of ultra-lean ground beef contains 7 grams of fat; 3 ounces of cooked lean ground beef contains about 14 grams of fat.

ITALIAN SPAGHETTI

Exchanges: 1 Starch, 1 Medium-Fat Meat, 1 Vegetable

Serving Size: 1 cup	**Calories:** 250
Carbohydrate: 28 gm	**Fiber:** 3 gm
Protein: 15 gm	**Sodium:** 302 mg
Fat: 9 gm	**Cholesterol:** 32 mg

INGREDIENTS:

½ pound lean ground beef
½ small onion, chopped
⅔ cup water
½ cup chopped tomato
⅓ cup tomato paste
2½ teaspoons Italian
   seasoning

½ teaspoon onion powder
¼ teaspoon garlic powder
¼ teaspoon dried oregano
⅛ teaspoon pepper
1 small bay leaf
2 cups cooked spaghetti
   (cooked without salt or fat)

STEPS IN PREPARATION:

1. Cook ground beef and onion in a nonstick skillet over medium heat until meat is browned, stirring until meat crumbles. Drain and pat dry with paper towels.
2. Return meat mixture to skillet; add water and next 8 ingredients. Bring to a boil; reduce heat, and simmer, covered, 1 hour. Add more water if needed.
3. To serve, remove and discard bay leaf. Spoon ½ cup sauce over ½ cup cooked spaghetti.

Yield: 4 servings

STUFFED PEPPERS

Exchanges: 2 Starch, 1½ Medium-Fat Meat

Serving Size: 1 stuffed pepper
Carbohydrate: 34 gm
Protein: 15 gm
Fat: 9 gm

Calories: 273
Fiber: 3 gm
Sodium: 908 mg
Cholesterol: 33 mg

INGREDIENTS:

4 medium-size green peppers
½ pound lean ground beef
½ cup chopped onion
1 cup canned tomatoes, drained
1 cup cooked long-grain rice (cooked without salt or fat)
1 tablespoon Worcestershire sauce

½ teaspoon Italian seasoning
¼ teaspoon salt
Dash of pepper
¼ cup soft breadcrumbs
Vegetable cooking spray
1 cup canned tomato sauce

STEPS IN PREPARATION:

1. Slice off stem end of peppers; remove and discard seeds and membranes. Blanch peppers 5 to 10 minutes in boiling water. Drain.
2. Cook ground beef and onion in a nonstick skillet over medium heat until meat is browned, stirring until meat crumbles. Drain and pat dry with paper towels.
3. Return meat mixture to skillet. Add tomatoes; cook until liquid evaporates.
4. Remove from heat; stir in rice and next 4 ingredients.
5. Spoon ½-cup portions of rice mixture into peppers; sprinkle evenly with breadcrumbs. Place peppers in a baking dish coated with cooking spray. Bake at 350° for 20 minutes or until lightly browned.
6. Heat tomato sauce; spoon ¼ cup sauce over each pepper.

Yield: 4 servings

GREEN PEPPER CASSEROLE

Exchanges: 1 Medium-Fat Meat, 1 Vegetable

Serving Size: ⅔ cup	**Calories:** 117
Carbohydrate: 6 gm	**Fiber:** 2 gm
Protein: 9 gm	**Sodium:** 30 mg
Fat: 6 gm	**Cholesterol:** 53 mg

INGREDIENTS:

½ pound ground chuck
Vegetable cooking spray
3 medium-size green peppers, finely chopped
2 medium onions, finely chopped
2 tablespoons chopped green onions

1 egg, lightly beaten
2 tablespoons minced fresh parsley
½ teaspoon dried thyme
¼ teaspoon pepper
¼ teaspoon garlic powder
⅛ teaspoon ground cloves
⅛ teaspoon ground allspice

STEPS IN PREPARATION:

1. Cook ground chuck in a Dutch oven over medium heat until browned, stirring until meat crumbles. Drain and pat dry with paper towels. Set meat aside.
2. Wipe Dutch oven with a paper towel; coat with cooking spray, and place over low heat until hot.
3. Add green pepper, onion, and green onions; sauté 5 minutes or until vegetables are tender. Return meat to Dutch oven. Add egg and remaining ingredients, stirring well.
4. Spoon mixture into a shallow 2-quart casserole coated with cooking spray. Bake at 375° for 20 minutes or until set.

Yield: 6 servings

CREOLE MEAT LOAF

Exchanges: 2 Medium-Fat Meat, 2 Vegetable

Serving Size: 1 slice	**Calories:** 206
Carbohydrate: 8 gm	**Fiber:** 1 gm
Protein: 17 gm	**Sodium:** 452 mg
Fat: 12 gm	**Cholesterol:** 75 mg

INGREDIENTS:

1 pound ground chuck
½ cup chopped onion
½ cup skim milk
½ teaspoon dry mustard
½ teaspoon salt
1 egg, lightly beaten
Vegetable cooking spray
½ cup chopped green pepper

3 tablespoons chopped onion
1½ cups tomato juice
¾ cup sliced fresh
    mushrooms
2 tablespoons water
1 teaspoon cornstarch
¼ teaspoon dried thyme

STEPS IN PREPARATION:

1. Combine first 6 ingredients, stirring well. Shape into a loaf, and place in an 8½- x 4½- x 3-inch loafpan coated with cooking spray. Bake at 350° for 1 hour. Cool in pan 10 minutes.
2. Coat a medium skillet with cooking spray; place over low heat until hot. Add green pepper and 3 tablespoons onion; sauté 2 to 3 minutes or until tender.
3. Remove from heat; add tomato juice and mushrooms.
4. Combine water, cornstarch, and thyme, stirring to blend; add to skillet, and bring to a boil. Boil, stirring constantly, 1 minute or until thickened and bubbly.
5. Invert meat loaf onto a serving platter, and spoon tomato juice mixture over meat loaf. To serve, cut meat loaf into 6 slices.

Yield: 6 servings

LASAGNA

Exchanges: 1 Starch, 2 Medium-Fat Meat

Serving Size: $^{1}/_{12}$ recipe
Carbohydrate: 17 gm
Protein: 16 gm
Fat: 8 gm

Calories: 205
Fiber: 2 gm
Sodium: 333 mg
Cholesterol: 45 mg

INGREDIENTS:

1 pound ground chuck
½ cup water
1 (16-ounce) can stewed tomatoes, undrained
2 teaspoons dried Italian seasoning
1 clove garlic, minced
1 (8-ounce) package whole wheat lasagna noodles
1 (10-ounce) package frozen chopped spinach

1 cup 1% low-fat cottage cheese
2 tablespoons grated Parmesan cheese
1 tablespoon dried parsley flakes
1 teaspoon dried oregano
Vegetable cooking spray
1 cup (4 ounces) shredded low-fat process American cheese

STEPS IN PREPARATION:

1. Cook ground chuck in a medium skillet over medium heat until browned, stirring until meat crumbles. Drain and pat dry with paper towels. Wipe skillet with a paper towel.
2. Return meat to skillet, and stir in water and next 3 ingredients. Cover and bring to a boil. Reduce heat, and simmer 20 minutes.
3. Cook noodles according to package directions, omitting salt and fat. Drain well, and set aside.
4. Cook spinach according to package directions, omitting salt and fat. Drain well, and squeeze excess moisture from spinach. Combine spinach and next 4 ingredients, stirring well.
5. Place half of noodles in a 13- x 9- x 2-inch baking dish coated with cooking spray. Top with half of spinach mixture, half of American cheese, and half of meat mixture.
6. Repeat layers with remaining noodles, spinach mixture, American cheese, and meat mixture. Bake at 350° for 30 minutes. Let stand 10 minutes before serving.

Yield: 12 servings

SIX-LAYER BEEF DINNER

Exchanges: 1 Starch, 1½ Medium-Fat Meat

Serving Size: ¾ cup
Carbohydrate: 19 gm
Protein: 12 gm
Fat: 8 gm

Calories: 202
Fiber: 3 gm
Sodium: 139 mg
Cholesterol: 32 mg

INGREDIENTS:

1 pound ground chuck
4 medium-size round red
   potatoes, peeled and cut
   into ¼-inch slices
2 large carrots, scraped and
   cut into ¼-inch slices
1 large onion, cut into ¼-inch
   slices

1 medium-size green pepper,
   cut into ¼-inch slices
1 (16-ounce) can whole
   tomatoes, undrained and
   chopped
¼ teaspoon pepper
⅛ teaspoon dried basil

STEPS IN PREPARATION:

1. Cook ground chuck in a large ovenproof skillet over medium heat until meat is browned, stirring until meat crumbles. Drain and pat dry with paper towels. Wipe skillet with a paper towel.
2. Return meat to skillet; layer potato and next 4 ingredients over meat. Sprinkle with ¼ teaspoon pepper and basil. Cover and bake at 350° for 45 minutes. Serve warm.

Yield: 8 servings

You don't have to give up beef if you are trying to lower your blood cholesterol. The American Heart Association guidelines allow up to 6 ounces of lean cooked meat, fish, or poultry each day. A 3-ounce serving of lean beef contains an acceptable level of saturated fat and dietary cholesterol when all visible fat is trimmed.

SWEET-AND-SOUR BEEF AND CABBAGE

Exchanges: 2 Medium-Fat Meat, 1 Vegetable

Serving Size: 1 cup	**Calories:** 192
Carbohydrate: 9 gm	**Fiber:** trace
Protein: 11 gm	**Sodium:** 458 mg
Fat: 2 gm	**Cholesterol:** 44 mg

INGREDIENTS:

1½ pounds ground chuck
½ cup chopped onion
½ cup sliced celery
½ cup chopped green pepper
2 tablespoons dried parsley
  flakes
¾ teaspoon salt

¼ teaspoon garlic powder
1 medium head cabbage,
  cored and cut into 6 wedges
½ cup tomato sauce
¼ cup vinegar
3 tablespoons granulated
  brown sugar substitute

STEPS IN PREPARATION:

1. Cook first 4 ingredients in a large nonstick skillet over medium heat until meat is browned and vegetables are tender, stirring until meat crumbles. Drain and pat dry with paper towels. Wipe skillet with a paper towel.
2. Return meat mixture to skillet, and sprinkle with parsley, salt, and garlic powder. Arrange cabbage over meat mixture.
3. Combine tomato sauce, vinegar, and brown sugar substitute, stirring well.
4. Pour tomato sauce mixture over cabbage and meat mixture; cover and bring to a boil. Reduce heat, and simmer 15 to 20 minutes or until thoroughly heated. Serve immediately.

Yield: 9 servings

POLYNESIAN BEEF KEBABS

Exchanges: 3½ Lean Meat, 1 Starch, 1 Fruit, 1 Vegetable

Serving Size: ⅙ of recipe
Carbohydrate: 34 gm
Protein: 31 gm
Fat: 8 gm

Calories: 331
Fiber: 5 gm
Sodium: 1068 mg
Cholesterol: 77 mg

INGREDIENTS:

1½ pounds boneless sirloin
      steak
½ cup dry sherry
½ cup low-sodium soy sauce
3 tablespoons sugar
3 tablespoons white vinegar
½ teaspoon salt
½ teaspoon garlic powder
½ teaspoon pepper
2 small red onions, each cut
      into 8 wedges

1 (8-ounce) package fresh
      mushrooms
2 medium green bell peppers,
      cut into 1-inch pieces
1 small peeled and cored
      pineapple, cut into 1-inch
      pieces
2 cups cherry tomatoes
Vegetable cooking spray

STEPS IN PREPARATION:

1. Trim fat from beef; cut beef into 1-inch cubes. Combine beef and
   next 7 ingredients in a large zip-top plastic bag; seal and marinate
   in refrigerator 2 to 24 hours, turning bag occasionally. Remove
   beef cubes from bag, reserving marinade.
2. Prepare grill or broiler.
3. Thread beef cubes, onion wedges, mushrooms, bell pepper pieces,
   and pineapple pieces alternately onto 12 (12-inch) skewers.
   Thread tomatoes separately onto 6 (12-inch) skewers.
4. Place beef-vegetable skewers on grill rack coated with cooking
   spray; cover and grill 10 minutes or until beef is desired degree of
   doneness, turning and basting occasionally with reserved marinade. Grill tomato skewers 2 minutes or until thoroughly heated.
5. Serve over cooked rice, if desired.

Yield: 6 servings

Note: See the Starch List on page 16 for exchange value of rice.

SLICED STEAK AU JUS

Exchanges: 2 Lean Meat

Serving Size: 2 ounces
Carbohydrate: 1 gm
Protein: 14 gm
Fat: 2 gm

Calories: 81
Fiber: 0 gm
Sodium: 140 mg
Cholesterol: 37 mg

INGREDIENTS:

1¾ pounds lean top round steak
Vegetable cooking spray
1 (3-ounce) can sliced mushrooms, drained
1 tablespoon Worcestershire sauce
1 tablespoon lemon juice
½ teaspoon salt
Dash of pepper
1 garlic clove, minced

STEPS IN PREPARATION:

1. Cut steak into ¼-inch slices; arrange slices in a shallow baking dish coated with cooking spray.
2. Sprinkle mushrooms and remaining ingredients over steak.
3. Cover and bake at 350° for 1 hour.
4. Uncover and bake an additional 15 minutes or to desired degree of doneness, basting occasionally.

Yield: 14 servings

Look for cuts of beef with "loin" or "round" in the name. They're among the leanest choices.

MARINATED STEAK

Exchanges: 2 Medium-Fat Meat

Serving Size: 2 ounces with sauce
Carbohydrate: 2 gm
Protein: 15 gm
Fat: 2 gm

Calories: 113
Fiber: 1 gm
Sodium: 261 mg
Cholesterol: 39 mg

INGREDIENTS:

1½ teaspoons Worcestershire
   sauce
4 (2½-ounce) lean round
   steaks
½ teaspoon garlic salt
½ teaspoon instant minced
   onion

½ teaspoon pepper
½ cup dry white wine
1 cup water
1 (3-ounce) can sliced
   mushrooms, drained

STEPS IN PREPARATION:

1. Spoon Worcestershire sauce over both sides of steaks. Sprinkle steaks with garlic salt, onion, and pepper. Cover and chill 1 hour.
2. Cook steaks in a nonstick skillet over medium heat until meat is browned on both sides.
3. Pour wine over steaks. Cover and reduce heat; simmer 15 minutes.
4. Remove steaks to a serving platter, and keep warm.
5. Add water and mushrooms to skillet; boil, uncovered, 10 minutes or until gravy is reduced to about ½ cup, stirring frequently. Spoon gravy over steaks, and serve.

Yield: 4 servings

Alcohol evaporates at 172°F, so when you use liqueurs, wines, and spirits in cooking, most of the alcohol evaporates, leaving only the flavor behind. However, the amount of alcohol that evaporates depends on the type of heat applied, the source of the alcohol (wine versus distilled spirits), and the cooking time.

STEAK DELUXE

Exchanges: ½ Starch, 2 Medium-Fat Meat

Serving Size: 2 ounces with sauce
Carbohydrate: 5 gm
Protein: 17 gm
Fat: 3 gm

Calories: 116
Fiber: 1 gm
Sodium: 190 mg
Cholesterol: 42 mg

INGREDIENTS:

1 pound lean round steak
2 tablespoons all-purpose flour
1 teaspoon reduced-calorie margarine
Vegetable cooking spray
1¼ cups cooked tomato
1 tablespoon granulated brown sugar substitute

2 teaspoons Worcestershire sauce
½ teaspoon celery salt
½ teaspoon vinegar
¼ teaspoon dried thyme
⅛ teaspoon garlic powder
⅛ teaspoon pepper
½ medium onion, sliced

STEPS IN PREPARATION:

1. Lightly dredge steak in flour.
2. Melt margarine in a nonstick skillet. Add steak, and cook over medium heat until steak is browned on both sides.
3. Transfer steak to a 13- x 9- x 2-inch baking dish coated with cooking spray.
4. Combine tomato and remaining ingredients; pour over steak. Cover; bake at 300° for 2½ hours. Uncover and bake an additional 15 minutes or until liquid is thickened.

Yield: 6 servings

SWISS STEAK

Exchanges: 3 Lean Meat, 2 Vegetable

Serving Size: ⅙ recipe
Carbohydrate: 7 gm
Protein: 27 gm
Fat: 5 gm

Calories: 188
Fiber: 1 gm
Sodium: 396 mg
Cholesterol: 70 mg

INGREDIENTS:

1½ pounds lean round steak, trimmed and cut into 6 pieces
1 tablespoon reduced-calorie margarine, melted
1 (16-ounce) can stewed tomatoes, undrained
1 small onion, sliced
1 stalk celery, sliced
1 medium carrot, scraped and thinly sliced
1 teaspoon Worcestershire sauce
1 tablespoon all-purpose flour
½ teaspoon salt
¼ cup water

STEPS IN PREPARATION:

1. Place each piece of steak between two sheets of heavy-duty plastic wrap, and flatten to ¼-inch thickness, using a meat mallet or rolling pin.
2. Cook meat in margarine in a large skillet over medium heat until both sides are browned. Drain and pat dry with paper towels.
3. Return meat to skillet; add stewed tomatoes and next 4 ingredients. Cover and cook over low heat 1 hour and 15 minutes or until meat is tender. Transfer meat to a serving platter, and keep warm.
4. Skim excess fat from tomato mixture. Combine flour and salt; add water, and stir until well blended. Stir into tomato mixture. Cook over medium heat 2 minutes or until thickened and bubbly, stirring frequently. Remove tomato mixture from heat; spoon over meat.

Yield: 6 servings

STIR-FRIED BEEF

Exchanges: 1 Lean Meat, 1 Vegetable

Serving Size: ½ cup
Carbohydrate: 6 gm
Protein: 11 gm
Fat: 1 gm

Calories: 81
Fiber: 1 gm
Sodium: 381 mg
Cholesterol: 24 mg

INGREDIENTS:

1 pound lean boneless top round steak, trimmed
⅔ cup water
¼ cup chopped onion
3 tablespoons reduced-sodium soy sauce
1 teaspoon beef-flavored bouillon granules
1 teaspoon Worcestershire sauce
½ teaspoon salt

⅛ teaspoon pepper
1 clove garlic, minced
2 cups cauliflower flowerets
2 medium carrots, scraped and diagonally sliced
Vegetable cooking spray
1 cup sliced fresh mushrooms
1 (6-ounce) package frozen snow pea pods, thawed
¼ cup water
1 tablespoon cornstarch

STEPS IN PREPARATION:

1. Partially freeze steak; slice diagonally across grain into ¼-inch strips. Set aside.
2. Combine ⅔ cup water and next 7 ingredients. Add steak, stirring to coat. Cover and chill 1 hour. Drain steak, reserving marinade.
3. Cook cauliflower and carrot in boiling water to cover 3 minutes; drain and set aside.
4. Coat a wok or large skillet with cooking spray; heat at medium-high (375°) 2 minutes. Add steak; stir-fry 3 minutes. Add mushrooms; stir-fry 1 minute. Add snow peas, carrot, and cauliflower; stir-fry 2 minutes or until vegetables are crisp-tender.
5. Combine reserved marinade, ¼ cup water, and cornstarch, stirring to blend. Pour over steak mixture, and stir-fry until thickened.
6. Serve over cooked rice (cooked without salt or fat), if desired.

Yield: 12 servings

Note: See the Starch List on page 16 for exchange value of rice.

BEEF STEW

Exchanges: 2 Starch, 2 Lean Meat, 1 Vegetable

Serving Size: 1 cup
Carbohydrate: 31 gm
Protein: 22 gm
Fat: 3 gm

Calories: 240
Fiber: 5 gm
Sodium: 887 mg
Cholesterol: 45 mg

INGREDIENTS:

1 pound lean beef, cubed
2 tablespoons Worcestershire
   sauce
½ teaspoon salt
¼ teaspoon dried oregano
⅛ teaspoon ground allspice
1 beef bouillon cube
2 cups boiling water

1 cup canned tomatoes,
   undrained
4 medium baking potatoes,
   cubed
3 medium carrots, sliced
3 small onions, quartered
1 (10-ounce) package frozen
   English peas

STEPS IN PREPARATION:

1. Marinate beef in Worcestershire sauce 4 hours.
2. Cook beef in a nonstick skillet over medium heat until browned
   on all sides. Add salt, oregano, and allspice.
3. Dissolve bouillon cube in boiling water; add to beef mixture. Add
   tomatoes, and cook over low heat 1½ to 2 hours or until meat is
   tender.
4. Add potato, carrot, and onion; cook 30 minutes.
5. Add peas; cook an additional 15 minutes or until vegetables are
   tender.

Yield: 6 servings

POT ROAST WITH VEGETABLES

Exchanges: 1 Starch, 3 Medium-Fat Meat

Serving Size: ⅙ recipe
Carbohydrate: 19 gm
Protein: 22 gm
Fat: 12 gm

Calories: 269
Fiber: 3 gm
Sodium: 195 mg
Cholesterol: 60 mg

INGREDIENTS:

1 pound lean boneless chuck roast, trimmed
Vegetable cooking spray
¼ cup water
¼ teaspoon salt
⅛ teaspoon pepper
2 medium onions, peeled and sliced

2 stalks celery, sliced
4 large carrots, scraped and sliced
2 medium-size red round potatoes, peeled and cubed

STEPS IN PREPARATION:

1. Cook roast over medium heat in a small Dutch oven coated with cooking spray until browned on all sides. Add water and next 4 ingredients. Cover and bake at 350° for 1 hour and 15 minutes.
2. Add carrot and potato; bake an additional hour or until meat and vegetables are tender.
3. Transfer meat and vegetables to a serving platter; cut roast into 2-ounce slices.

Yield: 6 servings

VEAL PARMIGIANA

Exchanges: 2 Lean Meat, 1 Vegetable

Serving Size: ⅙ recipe
Carbohydrate: 6 gm
Protein: 17 gm
Fat: 5 gm

Calories: 145
Fiber: 1 gm
Sodium: 555 mg
Cholesterol: 87 mg

INGREDIENTS:

1 egg, lightly beaten
½ teaspoon salt
¼ teaspoon pepper
¼ cup soft breadcrumbs
1 tablespoon grated
  Parmesan cheese

1 pound thin veal cutlets, cut
  into 6 pieces
Vegetable cooking spray
1 (8-ounce) can tomato sauce
2 (1-ounce) slices part-skim
  mozzarella cheese

STEPS IN PREPARATION:

1. Combine egg, salt, and pepper; beat with a wire whisk until blended. Combine breadcrumbs and Parmesan cheese in a shallow dish, stirring well. Dip veal into egg mixture, and dredge in breadcrumb mixture.
2. Cook veal over medium heat in a large skillet coated with cooking spray until lightly browned on both sides.
3. Transfer veal to a shallow baking dish coated with cooking spray. Pour tomato sauce over veal. Bake at 350° for 15 minutes. Top with cheese slices, and bake an additional 5 minutes. Serve immediately.

Yield: 6 servings

Because veal comes from young animals, it does not have the marbling (fat) that is found in other good cuts of meat. Most cuts of veal are considered lean, with the leg, shoulder, loin, and sirloin being the leanest.

VEAL SCALLOPINI

Exchanges: 2 Medium-Fat Meat, 1 Vegetable

Serving Size: ½ cup
Carbohydrate: 5 gm
Protein: 15 gm
Fat: 5 gm

Calories: 120
Fiber: 1 gm
Sodium: 523 mg
Cholesterol: 54 mg

INGREDIENTS:

½ cup chopped onion
¼ cup chopped green pepper
1 tablespoon reduced-calorie margarine, melted
1 pound veal cutlets, sliced into thin strips
1 cup canned tomato sauce

1 cup water
¼ teaspoon salt
¼ teaspoon dried thyme
⅛ teaspoon pepper
½ cup (2 ounces) shredded low-fat process American cheese

STEPS IN PREPARATION:

1. Sauté onion and green pepper in margarine in a nonstick skillet until tender; remove from skillet, and set aside.
2. Place veal in skillet, and cook over medium heat until browned on both sides.
3. Add tomato sauce and next 4 ingredients. Return onion and green pepper to skillet. Cover; simmer 15 minutes.
4. Remove from heat, and sprinkle with cheese.
5. Serve over spaghetti noodles (cooked without salt or fat), if desired.

Yield: 6 servings

Note: See the Starch List on page 16 for exchange value of noodles.

PORK CHOPS WITH APPLES

Exchanges: 3 Lean Meat, 1 Fruit

Serving Size: 1 chop with apple
Carbohydrate: 17 gm
Protein: 26 gm
Fat: 9 gm

Calories: 253
Fiber: 2 gm
Sodium: 363 mg
Cholesterol: 72 mg

INGREDIENTS:

4 (4-ounce) lean boneless
  center-cut pork chops
1 medium onion, chopped
Vegetable cooking spray
1¼ cups water
1 teaspoon chicken-flavored
  bouillon granules

¼ teaspoon pepper
3 medium cooking apples,
  peeled and sliced
½ teaspoon ground cinnamon

STEPS IN PREPARATION:

1. Cook pork chops and onion in a large skillet coated with cooking spray over medium heat until pork is lightly browned.
2. Combine water, bouillon granules, and pepper, stirring until granules dissolve; add to skillet.
3. Cover and bring to a boil. Reduce heat, and simmer 20 minutes. Skim off fat.
4. Add apple slices and cinnamon to skillet. Cover and simmer 15 minutes or until pork is tender.

Yield: 4 servings

PORK CHOP DINNER

Exchanges: 2 Starch, 3 Medium-Fat Meat

Serving Size: 1 chop with rice
Carbohydrate: 29 gm
Protein: 24 gm
Fat: 11 gm

Calories: 319
Fiber: 2 gm
Sodium: 1047 mg
Cholesterol: 69 mg

INGREDIENTS:

4 (6-ounce) lean center-cut
   pork chops (½ inch thick)
¼ cup chopped onion
¼ cup chopped green pepper
1½ cups canned tomatoes
½ cup long-grain rice,
   uncooked

1 teaspoon salt
¼ teaspoon dry mustard
⅛ teaspoon ground allspice
⅛ teaspoon pepper

STEPS IN PREPARATION:

1. Cook pork chops in a nonstick skillet over medium heat until lightly browned. Drain and pat dry with paper towels. Set chops aside.
2. Sauté onion and green pepper in skillet until tender.
3. Combine tomatoes and remaining ingredients; add to skillet.
4. Place pork chops on top of mixture in skillet. Cover; simmer 30 minutes or until rice is tender.

Yield: 4 servings

CREOLE PORK CHOPS

Exchanges: 2 Medium-Fat Meat, 2 Vegetable

Serving Size: 1 chop with sauce	**Calories:** 201
Carbohydrate: 9 gm	**Fiber:** 2 gm
Protein: 20 gm	**Sodium:** 555 mg
Fat: 10 gm	**Cholesterol:** 60 mg

INGREDIENTS:

4 (3-ounce) lean boneless
  pork chops
1 (16-ounce) can crushed
  tomatoes
⅓ cup chopped onion
¼ cup chopped green pepper

¼ cup chopped celery
½ teaspoon salt
½ teaspoon hot sauce
¼ teaspoon dried oregano
1 bay leaf

STEPS IN PREPARATION:

1. Cook chops in a nonstick skillet over medium heat until lightly browned. Drain and pat dry with paper towels.
2. Return chops to skillet. Add tomatoes and remaining ingredients; cover and simmer 1 hour or until chops are tender.
3. To serve, remove and discard bay leaf. Spoon sauce evenly over chops.

Yield: 4 servings

SWEET-AND-SOUR PORK

Exchanges: 1 Lean Meat, 1 Vegetable

Serving Size: ½ cup
Carbohydrate: 8 gm
Protein: 11 gm
Fat: 2 gm

Calories: 97
Fiber: trace
Sodium: 458 mg
Cholesterol: 44 mg

INGREDIENTS:

1½ cups fat-free chicken broth, divided
1 tablespoon cornstarch
1 tablespoon all-purpose flour
½ teaspoon salt
1 egg
1 pound lean boneless pork, trimmed and cubed
Vegetable cooking spray
½ cup chopped carrot

1 medium-size green pepper, chopped
1 clove garlic, minced
⅓ cup red wine vinegar
2 tablespoons reduced-sodium soy sauce
1 tablespoon cornstarch
¼ cup water
Sugar substitute to equal ¾ cup sugar*

STEPS IN PREPARATION:

1. Combine ¼ cup broth, 1 tablespoon cornstarch, and next 3 ingredients; beat with a wire whisk. Dip pork cubes into mixture.
2. Coat a skillet with cooking spray; place over medium heat until hot. Add pork; cook 5 minutes. Remove pork; drain.
3. Wipe skillet with a paper towel; coat skillet with cooking spray. Add carrot, pepper, and garlic; sauté until tender. Stir in remaining 1¼ cups broth, vinegar, and soy sauce.
4. Dissolve 1 tablespoon cornstarch in water. Stir into vegetable mixture, and bring to a boil. Reduce heat, and simmer, stirring constantly, 1 to 2 minutes or until vegetable mixture is thickened. Stir in pork and sugar substitute. Cover and simmer until pork is tender.
5. Serve over cooked rice (cooked without salt or fat), if desired.

Yield: 10 servings

Note: See the Starch List on page 16 for exchange value of rice.

*See the sugar substitution chart on page 354.

HAM AND CORN CASSEROLE

Exchanges: 2 Starch, 2 Medium-Fat Meat

Serving Size: ¾ cup
Carbohydrate: 29 gm
Protein: 17 gm
Fat: 9 gm

Calories: 256
Fiber: 2 gm
Sodium: 1203 mg
Cholesterol: 30 mg

INGREDIENTS:

3 tablespoons all-purpose flour
1½ cups skim milk, divided
3 tablespoons reduced-calorie margarine
2 cups cubed lean cooked ham
¼ cup chopped onion
¼ cup chopped green pepper
½ teaspoon dry mustard
¼ teaspoon salt

¼ teaspoon Worcestershire sauce
⅛ teaspoon pepper
1 (20-ounce) can whole kernel corn, drained
Vegetable cooking spray
1 cup soft breadcrumbs
1 cup (4 ounces) shredded low-fat process American cheese

STEPS IN PREPARATION:

1. Combine flour and ½ cup milk; stir until smooth. Combine flour mixture, remaining 1 cup milk, and margarine in a small saucepan; stir well. Cook over medium heat, stirring constantly, until mixture is thickened and bubbly.
2. Stir in ham and next 7 ingredients.
3. Spoon mixture into a 1½-quart casserole coated with cooking spray. Top with breadcrumbs and cheese. Bake at 375° for 25 minutes or until bubbly.

Yield: 8 servings

BAKED HAM WITH PINEAPPLE

Exchanges: 2 Lean Meat, ½ Fruit

Serving Size: ¹⁄₁₂ recipe	**Calories:** 122
Carbohydrate: 4 gm	**Fiber:** trace
Protein: 16 gm	**Sodium:** 910 mg
Fat: 4 gm	**Cholesterol:** 40 mg

INGREDIENTS:

1 (2-pound) fully cooked boneless smoked ham
20 whole cloves
4 slices canned pineapple in juice, drained
½ cup sugar-free ginger ale
1 teaspoon ground cinnamon

STEPS IN PREPARATION:

1. Remove and discard casing from ham. Score top of ham in a diamond design, and stud with cloves.
2. Place ham in a shallow baking dish, and arrange pineapple slices over ham. Pour ginger ale over ham, and sprinkle pineapple slices evenly with cinnamon. Bake at 325° for 25 to 30 minutes or until thoroughly heated.
3. To serve, cut into 12 slices.

Yield: 12 servings

Reduced-fat cooked hams are now available. Look for them in the meat section of your local supermarket.

Poultry

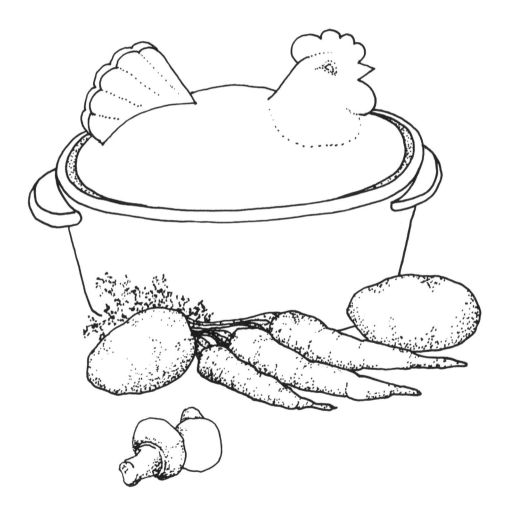

CHICKEN SALAD

Exchanges: 2 Lean Meat, 2 Vegetable

Serving Size: ¾ cup	**Calories:** 118
Carbohydrate: 10 gm	**Fiber:** 1 gm
Protein: 15 gm	**Sodium:** 796 mg
Fat: 2 gm	**Cholesterol:** 36 mg

INGREDIENTS:

2 cups diced cooked chicken (skinned before cooking and cooked without salt)
1 cup finely chopped celery
¾ cup reduced-calorie mayonnaise
⅔ cup chopped onion
1 tablespoon chopped pimiento
1 teaspoon salt
1 teaspoon Worcestershire sauce
¼ teaspoon pepper
Lettuce leaves (optional)

STEPS IN PREPARATION:

1. Combine first 8 ingredients; stir well. Cover and chill.
2. Serve on lettuce leaves, if desired.

Yield: 6 servings

For every chicken breast half, you can count on getting about ½ cup of chopped or diced chicken.

CHICKEN CASSEROLE

Exchanges: 1 Lean Meat, 1 Vegetable

Serving Size: ½ cup
Carbohydrate: 6 gm
Protein: 14 gm
Fat: 4 gm

Calories: 120
Fiber: trace
Sodium: 367 mg
Cholesterol: 32 mg

INGREDIENTS:

4 (3-ounce) skinned chicken breast halves
4 cups water
Vegetable cooking spray
¼ teaspoon salt
¼ teaspoon pepper
½ cup skim milk
½ (8-ounce) carton plain low-fat yogurt
½ (10½-ounce) can cream of chicken soup, undiluted
5 unsalted crackers, crushed
1 teaspoon reduced-calorie margarine, melted

STEPS IN PREPARATION:

1. Combine chicken breast halves and water in a medium saucepan; cover and bring to a boil. Reduce heat, and simmer 15 to 20 minutes or until chicken is done; drain well. Remove chicken from bone; coarsely chop chicken.
2. Place chopped chicken in a 1-quart casserole coated with cooking spray, and sprinkle with salt and pepper.
3. Combine milk, yogurt, and soup in a medium bowl, stirring until well blended; spoon mixture evenly over chicken.
4. Combine crushed crackers and melted margarine, stirring well. Sprinkle cracker mixture evenly over top of casserole. Bake at 350° for 20 minutes or until thoroughly heated.

Yield: 6 servings

CHICKEN-CAULIFLOWER CASSEROLE

Exchanges: 1 Lean Meat, 1½ Vegetable

Serving Size: ¾ cup	**Calories:** 106
Carbohydrate: 8 gm	**Fiber:** 1 gm
Protein: 11 gm	**Sodium:** 296 mg
Fat: 3 gm	**Cholesterol:** 22 mg

INGREDIENTS:

1 (10-ounce) package frozen chopped cauliflower
½ cup coarsely chopped onion
½ cup water
1 cup skim milk
1 tablespoon cornstarch
1 teaspoon low-sodium chicken-flavored bouillon granules
½ teaspoon salt
¼ cup (1 ounce) shredded low-fat process American cheese
1 cup chopped cooked chicken (skinned before cooking and cooked without salt)
1 (4-ounce) jar diced pimiento, drained
Vegetable cooking spray

STEPS IN PREPARATION:

1. Combine cauliflower, onion, and water in a medium saucepan; cover and bring to a boil. Reduce heat, and simmer 5 minutes or until vegetables are tender. Drain well, and set aside.
2. Add milk, cornstarch, bouillon granules, and salt to saucepan, stirring with a wire whisk. Bring to a boil; reduce heat, and simmer, stirring constantly, until thickened and bubbly.
3. Add cheese; stir with wire whisk until cheese melts. Remove from heat.
4. Add cauliflower mixture, chicken, and pimiento to cheese sauce. Spoon mixture into a 1½-quart casserole coated with cooking spray. Bake at 325° for 20 minutes or until thoroughly heated.

Yield: 6 servings

CHICKEN AND RICE CASSEROLE

Exchanges: 1 Starch, 2 Medium-Fat Meat

Serving Size: ½ cup	**Calories:** 210
Carbohydrate: 21 gm	**Fiber:** 1 gm
Protein: 15 gm	**Sodium:** 839 mg
Fat: 7 gm	**Cholesterol:** 90 mg

INGREDIENTS:

1½ cups diced cooked chicken (skinned before cooking and cooked without salt)

1 cup cooked long-grain rice (cooked without salt or fat)

½ cup chopped celery

¼ cup nonfat mayonnaise

1 tablespoon lemon juice

2 hard-cooked eggs, chopped

1 (10¾-ounce) can cream of mushroom soup, undiluted

1 small onion, chopped

Vegetable cooking spray

¼ cup soft breadcrumbs

1 tablespoon dry butter substitute

STEPS IN PREPARATION:

1. Combine first 8 ingredients; stir well. Spoon mixture into a shallow 2-quart casserole coated with cooking spray.
2. Combine bread crumbs and butter substitute; sprinkle over top of casserole. Bake at 350°, uncovered, for 40 to 45 minutes or until bubbly.

Yield: 6 servings

CHICKEN TORTILLA CASSEROLE

Exchanges: 1 Starch, 2 Lean Meat

Serving Size: ⅙ recipe
Carbohydrate: 16 gm
Protein: 15 gm
Fat: 7 gm

Calories: 180
Fiber: 2 gm
Sodium: 796 mg
Cholesterol: 32 mg

INGREDIENTS:

2 (4-ounce) skinned, boned chicken breast halves
4 cups water
½ cup skim milk
½ cup chunky salsa
½ small onion, grated
½ (10½-ounce) can cream of chicken soup, undiluted

6 (6-inch) corn tortillas, cut into wedges
1 cup (4 ounces) shredded low-fat process American cheese
Vegetable cooking spray
1½ large canned green chiles, seeded and diced

STEPS IN PREPARATION:

1. Combine chicken and water in a small saucepan; cover and bring to a boil. Reduce heat, and simmer 20 minutes or until chicken is done; drain well. Chop chicken, and set aside.
2. Combine milk, salsa, onion, and soup, stirring to blend. Layer half each of tortillas, chicken, soup mixture, and cheese in a 1½-quart casserole coated with cooking spray. Sprinkle with chiles.
3. Repeat layers with remaining tortillas, chicken, soup mixture, and cheese. Cover and chill overnight.
4. Bake at 300° for 1 hour or until thoroughly heated. Divide into 6 equal portions, and serve warm.

Yield: 6 servings

CHICKEN AND VEGETABLE CASSEROLE

Exchanges: ½ Starch, 2 Medium-Fat Meat, 1 Vegetable

Serving Size: 1 cup
Carbohydrate: 7 gm
Protein: 24 gm
Fat: 3 gm

Calories: 168
Fiber: 0 gm
Sodium: 129 mg
Cholesterol: 28 mg

INGREDIENTS:

1 (10¾-ounce) can cream of mushroom soup, undiluted
¼ cup skim milk
1 teaspoon Worcestershire sauce
1 cup diced cooked chicken (skinned before cooking and cooked without salt)

1 cup cooked sliced okra
¼ cup chopped celery
¼ cup chopped green pepper
Vegetable cooking spray

STEPS IN PREPARATION:

1. Combine first 3 ingredients in a medium bowl.
2. Add chicken, okra, celery, and green pepper.
3. Spoon mixture into a 1-quart casserole coated with cooking spray. Bake at 350° for 20 minutes or until thoroughly heated.

Yield: 4 servings

BOMBAY CHICKEN

Exchanges: ½ Starch, 2 Lean Meat

Serving Size: ½ cup
Carbohydrate: 11 gm
Protein: 12 gm
Fat: 6 gm

Calories: 138
Fiber: 2 gm
Sodium: 300 mg
Cholesterol: 22 mg

INGREDIENTS:

1 teaspoon reduced-calorie margarine
¼ cup chopped almonds
2 teaspoons curry powder, divided
1 cup diced apple
½ cup chopped onion
½ cup sliced fresh mushrooms
1 tablespoon all-purpose flour

1 teaspoon chicken-flavored bouillon granules
1 cup boiling water
½ cup skim milk
1 tablespoon lemon juice
1 cup chopped cooked chicken (skinned before cooking and cooked without salt)

STEPS IN PREPARATION:

1. Melt margarine in a large skillet over medium heat; add almonds. Cook 10 minutes or until almonds are golden, stirring frequently. Sprinkle almonds with 1 teaspoon curry powder; toss lightly to coat. Drain almonds on paper towels.
2. Add apple, onion, and mushrooms to skillet; sauté 5 minutes. Stir in remaining 1 teaspoon curry powder and flour. Cook over low heat 2 minutes, stirring frequently.
3. Dissolve bouillon granules in boiling water; add to skillet. Stir in milk and lemon juice. Cook over low heat, stirring constantly, 5 minutes or until thickened.
4. Add chicken; cook over low heat, stirring constantly, until thoroughly heated.

Yield: 5 servings

CURRIED CHICKEN

Exchanges: 2 Lean Meat, 1 Vegetable

Serving Size: ½ cup
Carbohydrate: 9 gm
Protein: 13 gm
Fat: 3 gm

Calories: 118
Fiber: 1 gm
Sodium: 209 mg
Cholesterol: 28 mg

INGREDIENTS:

1 large apple, chopped
¼ cup sliced green onions
1 tablespoon curry powder
1 tablespoon water
1 cup skim milk
2 tablespoons minced fresh parsley

½ (10¾-ounce) can cream of mushroom soup, undiluted
2 cups chopped cooked chicken (skinned before cooking and cooked without salt)
½ cup plain low-fat yogurt

STEPS IN PREPARATION:

1. Combine first 4 ingredients in a medium saucepan; cover and cook over medium heat until onions are tender.
2. Add milk, parsley, and soup, stirring well. Add chicken; cook 10 minutes.
3. Remove from heat, and stir in yogurt.
4. Serve over cooked rice (cooked without salt or fat), if desired.

Yield: 8 servings

Note: See the Starch List on page 16 for exchange value of rice.

CHICKEN CHOW MEIN

Exchanges: 1 Lean Meat, 1 Vegetable

Serving Size: ½ cup	**Calories:** 58
Carbohydrate: 5 gm	**Fiber:** 1 gm
Protein: 7 gm	**Sodium:** 340 mg
Fat: 1 gm	**Cholesterol:** 31 mg

INGREDIENTS:

Vegetable cooking spray
1½ cups chopped onion
1 cup sliced celery
½ cup chopped green pepper
2 cups chopped cooked chicken
(skinned before cooking and
cooked without salt)
1 (14-ounce) can Chinese-style
vegetables, drained

1 (4-ounce) can sliced
mushrooms, drained
¼ teaspoon ground cumin
1 tablespoon low-sodium
chicken-flavored bouillon
granules
3 cups water, divided
1 tablespoon cornstarch

STEPS IN PREPARATION:

1. Coat a large skillet with cooking spray; place over medium heat until hot. Add onion, celery, and green pepper; sauté 3 minutes or until vegetables are tender.
2. Stir in chicken and next 3 ingredients; cook over medium heat 1 minute.
3. Add bouillon granules and 2¾ cups water to chicken mixture. Cook over medium heat, stirring constantly, until granules dissolve.
4. Combine cornstarch and remaining ¼ cup water, stirring until smooth. Add cornstarch mixture to chicken mixture; cook over medium heat, stirring constantly, until thickened and bubbly.
5. Serve over cooked rice (cooked without salt or fat), if desired.

Yield: 14 servings

Note: See the Starch List on page 16 for exchange value of rice.

CHICKEN CACCIATORE

Exchanges: 1 Lean Meat, 2 Vegetable

Serving Size: 1 cup	**Calories:** 119
Carbohydrate: 12 gm	**Fiber:** 4 gm
Protein: 13 gm	**Sodium:** 412 mg
Fat: 3 gm	**Cholesterol:** 25 mg

INGREDIENTS:

1 tablespoon reduced-calorie margarine
½ pound skinned, boned chicken breast halves
½ cup chopped onion
½ cup chopped celery
1 clove garlic, minced
1 cup sliced fresh mushrooms
½ cup chopped fresh parsley
¼ cup chopped green pepper
1 teaspoon dried basil
1 teaspoon dried oregano
¼ teaspoon salt
¼ teaspoon black pepper
⅛ teaspoon ground red pepper
1 (28-ounce) can whole tomatoes, undrained and chopped

STEPS IN PREPARATION:

1. Melt margarine over low heat in a large skillet; add chicken, and cook until lightly browned. Chop chicken, and set aside.
2. Add onion, celery, and garlic to margarine in skillet; sauté until vegetables are tender.
3. Return chicken to skillet; add mushrooms and remaining ingredients. Cover and simmer 20 minutes.
4. Serve over cooked rice or noodles (cooked without salt or fat), if desired.

Yield: 5 servings

Note: See the Starch List on page 16 for exchange values of rice and noodles.

CHICKEN SPAGHETTI

Exchanges: 1 Starch, 2½ Lean Meat

Serving Size: 1 cup	**Calories:** 176
Carbohydrate: 14 gm	**Fiber:** trace
Protein: 20 gm	**Sodium:** 363 mg
Fat: 4 gm	**Cholesterol:** 44 mg

INGREDIENTS:

1½ pounds skinned, boned
   chicken breast halves
8 cups water
4 ounces spaghetti, uncooked
½ cup skim milk
½ teaspoon salt

¼ teaspoon pepper
½ (10¾-ounce) can cream of
   mushroom soup, undiluted
1 (2-ounce) jar sliced
   mushrooms, drained
Vegetable cooking spray

STEPS IN PREPARATION:

1. Combine chicken and water in a large skillet; cover and bring to a
   boil. Reduce heat, and simmer 15 to 20 minutes or until done;
   drain well. Chop chicken, and set aside.
2. Cook spaghetti according to package directions, omitting salt and
   fat; drain, and set aside.
3. Combine milk and next 3 ingredients, stirring to blend.
4. Layer spaghetti, chicken, soup mixture, and mushrooms in a
   13- x 9- x 2-inch baking dish coated with cooking spray. Bake at
   325° for 30 to 45 minutes or until thoroughly heated.

Yield: 8 servings

BAKED CHICKEN

Exchanges: 2 Lean Meat, 1½ Vegetable

Serving Size: 1 breast half
Carbohydrate: 8 gm
Protein: 18 gm
Fat: 2 gm

Calories: 128
Fiber: 2 gm
Sodium: 180 mg
Cholesterol: 43 mg

INGREDIENTS:

4 (3-ounce) skinned, boned chicken breast halves
Vegetable cooking spray
1 (12-ounce) can whole tomatoes, undrained and chopped

½ cup chopped green pepper
½ cup chopped onion
½ teaspoon garlic powder
¼ teaspoon dried basil
¼ teaspoon dried oregano
¼ teaspoon pepper

STEPS IN PREPARATION:

1. Arrange chicken breast halves in an 11- x 7- x 2-inch baking dish coated with cooking spray.
2. Combine tomato and remaining ingredients, stirring well; spoon over chicken in dish.
3. Cover and bake at 400° for 1 hour or until chicken is done.

Yield: 4 servings

A 3-ounce portion of skinned cooked dark meat chicken has twice the fat of a 3-ounce portion of skinned cooked white meat.

BAKED CHICKEN WITH RICE

Exchanges: 2 Starch, 2 Medium-Fat Meat

Serving Size: 1 breast half
Carbohydrate: 34 gm
Protein: 30 gm
Fat: 8 gm

Calories: 336
Fiber: 1 gm
Sodium: 1057 mg
Cholesterol: 67 mg

INGREDIENTS:

1 cup long-grain rice, uncooked
Vegetable cooking spray
1 (1-ounce) package onion soup mix, divided
6 (3-ounce) skinned, boned chicken breast halves

1 (10¾-ounce) can cream of mushroom soup, undiluted
1½ cups water
⅛ teaspoon pepper

STEPS IN PREPARATION:

1. Spread rice evenly in bottom of a 9-inch square baking dish coated with cooking spray. Sprinkle with one-fourth of onion soup mix.
2. Place chicken on top of rice. Add remaining onion soup mix.
3. Combine mushroom soup, water, and pepper. Pour mushroom soup mixture over chicken. Cover and bake at 325° for 2 hours or until chicken is done.

Yield: 6 servings

CREOLE CHICKEN

Exchanges: 2 Lean Meat, 2 Vegetable

Serving Size: 1 breast half	**Calories:** 103
Carbohydrate: 9 gm	**Fiber:** 2 gm
Protein: 13 gm	**Sodium:** 491 mg
Fat: 2 gm	**Cholesterol:** 29 mg

INGREDIENTS:

4 (3-ounce) skinned, boned chicken breast halves
Vegetable cooking spray
½ cup chopped celery
⅓ cup sliced onion
½ teaspoon salt
½ teaspoon dried thyme
⅛ teaspoon pepper
1 medium-size green pepper, cut into strips
1 (16-ounce) can crushed tomatoes

STEPS IN PREPARATION:

1. Place chicken breasts on rack of a broiler pan coated with cooking spray. Broil 5 inches from heat 10 minutes or until lightly browned, turning once.
2. Combine celery and remaining ingredients in a large nonstick skillet. Bring mixture to a boil; cover and cook over medium heat 10 minutes.
3. Add chicken; cover and reduce heat. Simmer 30 minutes or until chicken is tender.

Yield: 4 servings

CHICKEN DIJON

Exchanges: ½ Starch, 2 Lean Meat

Serving Size: 1 breast half	**Calories:** 133
Carbohydrate: 6 gm	**Fiber:** trace
Protein: 19 gm	**Sodium:** 194 mg
Fat: 3 gm	**Cholesterol:** 44 mg

INGREDIENTS:

¼ cup Dijon mustard
½ (8-ounce) carton plain
   nonfat yogurt
8 (3-ounce) skinned chicken
   breast halves

½ cup soft breadcrumbs
Vegetable cooking spray

STEPS IN PREPARATION:

1. Combine mustard and yogurt, stirring until well blended. Brush chicken breast halves evenly with yogurt mixture, and dredge in breadcrumbs.
2. Arrange chicken in a 13- x 9- x 2-inch baking dish coated with cooking spray. Cover and bake at 400° for 30 minutes.
3. Increase temperature to 450°. Bake, uncovered, for 15 minutes or until lightly browned.

Yield: 8 servings

HERBED CHICKEN

Exchanges: 2 Lean Meat

Serving Size: 1 breast half
Carbohydrate: trace
Protein: 12 gm
Fat: 2 gm

Calories: 64
Fiber: 0 gm
Sodium: 492 mg
Cholesterol: 29 mg

INGREDIENTS:

6 (4-ounce) skinned chicken
   breast halves
Vegetable cooking spray
2 teaspoons dried rosemary

½ teaspoon salt
¼ teaspoon pepper
2 chicken bouillon cubes
1 cup water

STEPS IN PREPARATION:

1. Place chicken in a shallow baking dish coated with cooking spray. Sprinkle with rosemary, salt, and pepper.
2. Crumble bouillon cubes between pieces of chicken.
3. Add water to baking dish.
4. Cover and bake at 350° for 1 hour or until chicken is done. Uncover and bake an additional 5 minutes or until chicken is lightly browned.

Yield: 6 servings

Cooking with herbs? Use finely chopped fresh herbs whenever possible for the best flavor. When substituting, use three times as much fresh herbs as dried herbs.

GRILLED MARINATED CHICKEN

Exchanges: 2 Lean Meat

Serving Size: 1 breast half	**Calories:** 108
Carbohydrate: 4 gm	**Fiber:** trace
Protein: 14 gm	**Sodium:** 240 mg
Fat: 3 gm	**Cholesterol:** 36 mg

INGREDIENTS:

6 (3-ounce) skinned chicken
  breast halves
Sugar substitute to equal ¼
  cup plus 2 tablespoons
  sugar*
3 tablespoons lemon juice

3 tablespoons vinegar
2 tablespoons reduced-calorie
  mayonnaise
½ teaspoon salt
½ teaspoon pepper
Vegetable cooking spray

STEPS IN PREPARATION:

1. Place chicken in a shallow dish.
2. Combine sugar substitute and next 5 ingredients, stirring well. Pour over chicken. Cover and marinate in refrigerator at least 1 hour.
3. Remove chicken from marinade, reserving marinade. Coat grill rack with cooking spray; place on grill over hot coals (400° to 500°). Place chicken on rack; grill, uncovered, for 45 minutes or until done. Turn and baste every 10 minutes with reserved marinade.

Yield: 6 servings

*See the sugar substitution chart on page 354.

OVEN-FRIED CHICKEN

Exchanges: ½ Starch, 3 Lean Meat

Serving Size: 1 breast half
Carbohydrate: 7 gm
Protein: 24 gm
Fat: 3 gm

Calories: 155
Fiber: 0 gm
Sodium: 129 mg
Cholesterol: 58 mg

INGREDIENTS:

1 cup crushed corn flakes cereal
¼ teaspoon paprika
¼ teaspoon onion powder
¼ teaspoon garlic powder
¼ teaspoon curry powder
4 (4-ounce) skinned chicken breast halves
4 teaspoons skim milk
Vegetable cooking spray

STEPS IN PREPARATION:

1. Combine first 5 ingredients in a shallow dish.
2. Dip chicken in milk, and dredge in cereal mixture.
3. Place chicken in a small baking dish coated with cooking spray. Bake at 350° for 20 to 30 minutes or until lightly browned.

Yield: 4 servings

Chicken with a crisp oven-fried coating and low-fat gravy offers a satisfying yet healthier alternative to pan- or deep-fried chicken.

SOY CHICKEN

Exchanges: ½ Starch, 3 Lean Meat

Serving Size: 1 breast half
Carbohydrate: 4 gm
Protein: 27 gm
Fat: 3 gm

Calories: 162
Fiber: 0 gm
Sodium: 1105 mg
Cholesterol: 66 mg

INGREDIENTS:

6 (4-ounce) skinned chicken
   breast halves
Dash of onion powder
Dash of garlic powder

⅓ cup soy sauce
⅓ cup Worcestershire sauce
⅓ cup vinegar
⅓ cup water

STEPS IN PREPARATION:

1. Sprinkle both sides of chicken with onion and garlic powders. Place chicken in a shallow baking dish.
2. Combine soy sauce and remaining ingredients. Pour soy sauce mixture over chicken.
3. Cover and chill at least 3 hours.
4. Bake, uncovered, at 350° 1 hour or until chicken is tender.

Yield: 6 servings

If you need to reduce sodium, use low-sodium soy sauce and low-sodium Worcestershire sauce instead of the regular products.

SQUASH MIX WITH CHICKEN

Exchanges: 1 Lean Meat, 2 Vegetable

Serving Size: 1 cup
Carbohydrate: 10 gm
Protein: 7 gm
Fat: 1 gm

Calories: 78
Fiber: 3 gm
Sodium: 311 mg
Cholesterol: 14 mg

INGREDIENTS:

½ cup chopped onion
½ cup sliced celery
1 teaspoon reduced-calorie
  margarine, melted
2½ cups sliced yellow squash
1 cup sliced zucchini
½ cup chopped cooked chicken
  (skinned before cooking and
  cooked without salt)

2 tablespoons water
½ teaspoon salt
½ teaspoon dried chervil
⅛ teaspoon ground red
  pepper
⅛ teaspoon black pepper

STEPS IN PREPARATION:

1. Sauté onion and celery in margarine in a large skillet until tender. Stir in squash and remaining ingredients. Cover and bring to a boil.
2. Reduce heat, and simmer 8 to 10 minutes or until vegetables are tender, stirring frequently.
3. Transfer mixture to a serving dish, and serve warm.

Yield: 4 servings

CHICKEN TOSTADA WITH SALSA

Exchanges: 1 Starch, 2 Lean Meat

Serving Size: 1 tortilla half	**Calories:** 172
Carbohydrate: 16 gm	**Fiber:** 1 gm
Protein: 14 gm	**Sodium:** 336 mg
Fat: 6 gm	**Cholesterol:** 31 mg

INGREDIENTS:

1 tablespoon vegetable oil
4 (8-inch) flour tortillas
3 cups shredded lettuce
2 medium tomatoes
¼ cup chopped green onions
2 cups shredded cooked chicken (skinned before cooking and cooked without salt)

¼ cup (1 ounce) shredded low-fat process American cheese
1 cup Salsa (see page 296)

STEPS IN PREPARATION:

1. Place oil in a large skillet, and place skillet over medium heat until oil is hot.
2. Add tortillas, one at a time, and cook 1 minute on each side or until thoroughly heated. Cut each tortilla in half.
3. Spoon lettuce evenly onto tortilla halves. Cut each tomato into 8 wedges, and arrange on lettuce. Sprinkle evenly with onions, and top evenly with shredded chicken and cheese. Spoon 2 tablespoons Salsa over each tortilla half.

Yield: 8 servings

CHICKEN CORDON BLEU

Exchanges: 3 Lean Meat, 1 Vegetable

Serving Size: 1 chicken roll
Carbohydrate: 7 gm
Protein: 21 gm
Fat: 8 gm

Calories: 192
Fiber: trace
Sodium: 398 mg
Cholesterol: 98 mg

INGREDIENTS:

4 (3-ounce) skinned, boned chicken breast halves
2 (1-ounce) slices lean cooked ham, cut in half
2 (1-ounce) slices low-fat process Swiss cheese, cut in half

1 egg, lightly beaten
2 tablespoons all-purpose flour
Vegetable cooking spray
⅓ cup chopped onion
¼ (10½-ounce) can cream of chicken soup, undiluted

STEPS IN PREPARATION:

1. Place chicken between 2 sheets of heavy-duty plastic wrap, and flatten to ¼-inch thickness using a meat mallet or rolling pin.
2. Place one slice each of ham and cheese in center of each chicken breast half. Roll up lengthwise, and secure with wooden picks.
3. Dip each chicken roll in egg, and dredge in flour. Place chicken rolls, seam side down, in a shallow baking dish coated with cooking spray. Bake at 350° for 20 minutes.
4. Combine onion and soup, stirring well. Spoon over chicken, and bake at 350° for 15 minutes or until chicken is done.

Yield: 4 servings

CHICKEN DIVAN

Exchanges: 2 Lean Meat, 1 Vegetable

Serving Size: 1 cup	**Calories:** 113
Carbohydrate: 4 gm	**Fiber:** 1 gm
Protein: 17 gm	**Sodium:** 224 mg
Fat: 3 gm	**Cholesterol:** 39 mg

INGREDIENTS:

8 (3-ounce) skinned, boned chicken breast halves
8 cups water
1 (10-ounce) package frozen chopped broccoli, thawed
Vegetable cooking spray
¼ (10¾-ounce) can cream of chicken soup, undiluted
¼ (10¾-ounce) can cream of potato soup, undiluted
½ cup skim milk
1½ teaspoons lemon juice
2 tablespoons grated Parmesan cheese

STEPS IN PREPARATION:

1. Combine chicken and water in a large saucepan; cover and bring to a boil. Reduce heat, and simmer 20 minutes or until chicken is done; drain well. Chop chicken.
2. Place broccoli in a 2-quart baking dish coated with cooking spray; top with chicken.
3. Combine soups, milk, and lemon juice, stirring to blend; pour over chicken and broccoli. Sprinkle with cheese. Bake at 350° for 25 minutes or until thoroughly heated.

Yield: 8 servings

CHICKEN AND DUMPLINGS

Exchanges: 1 Starch, 2 Medium-Fat Meat

Serving Size: ¾ cup
Carbohydrate: 18 gm
Protein: 14 gm
Fat: 9 gm

Calories: 213
Fiber: 1 gm
Sodium: 371 mg
Cholesterol: 33 mg

INGREDIENTS:

1 (3-pound) broiler-fryer, skinned
1½ cups water
¼ cup chopped celery
¼ cup chopped onion
¼ teaspoon salt

1 cup all-purpose flour
1 teaspoon baking powder
½ teaspoon salt
3 tablespoons vegetable shortening
¼ cup skim milk

STEPS IN PREPARATION:

1. Disjoint chicken; place in a large Dutch oven. Add water and next 3 ingredients; simmer 1 hour or until chicken is tender.
2. Combine flour, baking powder, and salt. Cut in shortening with a pastry blender. Add milk to make a stiff dough. Roll dough out to ⅛-inch thickness, and cut into 1-inch-square dumplings.
3. Remove chicken from bone; return chicken to chicken stock.
4. Bring stock to a boil; add dumplings. Cover, reduce heat, and simmer 8 to 10 minutes or until dumplings are done.

Yield: 6 servings

CHICKEN FLORENTINE WITH MUSHROOM SAUCE

Exchanges: 1 Starch, 3 Lean Meat

Serving Size: ½ recipe	**Calories:** 214
Carbohydrate: 16 gm	**Fiber:** 4 gm
Protein: 24 gm	**Sodium:** 594 mg
Fat: 7 gm	**Cholesterol:** 43 mg

INGREDIENTS:

2 (3-ounce) skinned, boned chicken breast halves
¼ cup chopped onion
Vegetable cooking spray
1 (10-ounce) package frozen chopped spinach, thawed
2 tablespoons shredded reduced-fat Swiss cheese
⅛ teaspoon ground nutmeg

½ cup sliced fresh mushrooms
½ cup skim milk
½ cup water
1 tablespoon reduced-calorie margarine, melted
½ teaspoon chicken-flavored bouillon granules

STEPS IN PREPARATION:

1. Place chicken between 2 sheets of heavy-duty plastic wrap, and flatten to ¼-inch thickness using a meat mallet or rolling pin. Set chicken aside.
2. Sauté onion in a large skillet coated with cooking spray. Remove from heat, and stir in spinach, cheese, and nutmeg.
3. Divide spinach mixture in half, and shape into mounds. Transfer mounds to an 11- x 7- x 2-inch baking dish coated with cooking spray. Top each portion with a chicken breast half. Bake at 350° for 25 minutes or until chicken is done.
4. Place mushrooms in skillet. Stir in milk and remaining ingredients, and bring to a boil; boil 6 minutes or until liquid is reduced and thickened, stirring frequently. Spoon sauce evenly over chicken, and serve warm.

Yield: 2 servings

SPINACH-CHICKEN ROLLS

Exchanges: 2 Lean Meat, 1 Vegetable

Serving Size: 1 chicken roll
Carbohydrate: 8 gm
Protein: 14 gm
Fat: 2 gm

Calories: 108
Fiber: 2 gm
Sodium: 276 mg
Cholesterol: 30 mg

INGREDIENTS:

1 small onion, chopped
¼ pound fresh mushrooms, chopped
Vegetable cooking spray
1 (10-ounce) package frozen chopped spinach, thawed
2 tablespoons grated Parmesan cheese
1 tablespoon chili sauce
½ teaspoon dried whole basil
¼ teaspoon salt

8 (3-ounce) skinned, boned chicken breast halves
1 (16-ounce) can whole tomatoes, drained and chopped
⅓ cup finely chopped onion
½ teaspoon dried Italian seasoning
¼ teaspoon pepper
1 clove garlic, crushed
2 tablespoons tomato sauce

STEPS IN PREPARATION:

1. Combine 1 chopped onion and mushrooms in a shallow 2-quart casserole coated with cooking spray. Cover and microwave at HIGH 4 minutes; drain.
2. Place spinach on paper towels, and squeeze until barely moist. Add spinach and next 4 ingredients to onion mixture.
3. Place chicken between 2 sheets of heavy-duty plastic wrap; flatten to ¼-inch thickness using a meat mallet. Place ¼ cup spinach mixture in center of each chicken piece. Roll up lengthwise; secure with wooden picks. Place in casserole coated with cooking spray.
4. Combine tomato and next 4 ingredients; spoon over chicken. Cover and microwave at HIGH 12 minutes, rotating dish after 5 minutes and rearranging rolls so that uncooked portions are to outside of dish.
5. Transfer chicken to a warm platter. Stir 2 tablespoons tomato sauce into liquid in dish. Cover and microwave at HIGH 2 minutes. Spoon over chicken.

Yield: 8 servings

CHICKEN LIVERS AND RICE

Exchanges: 1 Starch, 1 Medium-Fat Meat

Serving Size: ½ cup
Carbohydrate: 20 gm
Protein: 8 gm
Fat: 5 gm

Calories: 161
Fiber: 1 gm
Sodium: 559 mg
Cholesterol: 114 mg

INGREDIENTS:

3 tablespoons minced onion
2 teaspoons reduced-calorie margarine, melted
2 cups cooked rice (cooked without salt or fat)
½ pound chicken livers, cut into 1-inch pieces
2 tablespoons all-purpose flour

2 tablespoons reduced-calorie margarine, melted
½ cup skim milk
1 tablespoon chopped parsley
Dash of pepper
1 (10¾-ounce) can cream of chicken soup, undiluted
Vegetable cooking spray

STEPS IN PREPARATION:

1. Sauté onion in 2 teaspoons margarine in a medium saucepan until tender. Combine onion and rice; set aside.
2. Dredge chicken livers lightly in flour. Sauté livers in 2 tablespoons margarine in a nonstick skillet until browned on all sides.
3. Combine livers, rice mixture, milk, and next 3 ingredients; place mixture in a 1½-quart casserole coated with cooking spray. Bake at 375° for 30 minutes or until hot and bubbly.

Yield: 8 servings

TURKEY HASH

Exchanges: 1 Starch, 1 Medium-Fat Meat

Serving Size: ½ cup
Carbohydrate: 15 gm
Protein: 11 gm
Fat: 5 gm

Calories: 145
Fiber: 2 gm
Sodium: 503 mg
Cholesterol: 26 mg

INGREDIENTS:

¼ cup chopped onion
2 teaspoons reduced-calorie margarine, melted
1½ cups diced cooked potatoes
1 cup diced cooked turkey breast
⅔ cup cooked English peas

1 (10¾-ounce) can cream of celery soup, undiluted
Vegetable cooking spray
¼ cup (1 ounce) shredded low-fat process American cheese
¼ teaspoon paprika

STEPS IN PREPARATION:

1. Sauté onion in margarine in a nonstick skillet until tender. Add potato and next 3 ingredients.
2. Place mixture in a 1-quart casserole coated with cooking spray. Top with shredded cheese and paprika. Bake at 350° for 30 minutes or until thoroughly heated.

Yield: 6 servings

Store fresh uncooked turkey in its original package for up to three days in the refrigerator. If you don't plan to cook it within that time, freeze it as soon as possible to maintain optimum flavor. You can freeze turkey for up to three months.

TURKEY-STUFFED TOMATOES

Exchanges: 2 Lean Meat, 2 Vegetable

Serving Size: 1 stuffed tomato	**Calories:** 134
Carbohydrate: 11 gm	**Fiber:** 2 gm
Protein: 17 gm	**Sodium:** 433 mg
Fat: 3 gm	**Cholesterol:** 35 mg

INGREDIENTS:

6 medium tomatoes
½ teaspoon salt
1 cup skim milk
1 tablespoon all-purpose
  flour
1¾ cups chopped cooked
  turkey breast

½ cup chopped celery
¼ cup chopped green onions
¼ cup (1 ounce) shredded
  low-fat process American
  cheese
½ teaspoon salt
¼ teaspoon pepper

STEPS IN PREPARATION:

1. Cut tops from tomatoes; scoop out pulp, leaving shells intact. Reserve pulp for other uses. Sprinkle inside of tomato shells with ½ teaspoon salt, and invert on paper towels to drain.
2. Combine milk and flour in a small saucepan, stirring to blend. Bring to a boil; reduce heat to low, and cook, stirring constantly, until smooth and thickened.
3. Stir in turkey, celery, onions, and cheese. Sprinkle with remaining ½ teaspoon salt and pepper.
4. Spoon turkey mixture into tomato shells, and place shells in a 13- x 9- x 2-inch baking dish. Bake at 375° for 15 to 20 minutes or until thoroughly heated.

Yield: 6 servings

Rice, Pasta, and Starchy Vegetables

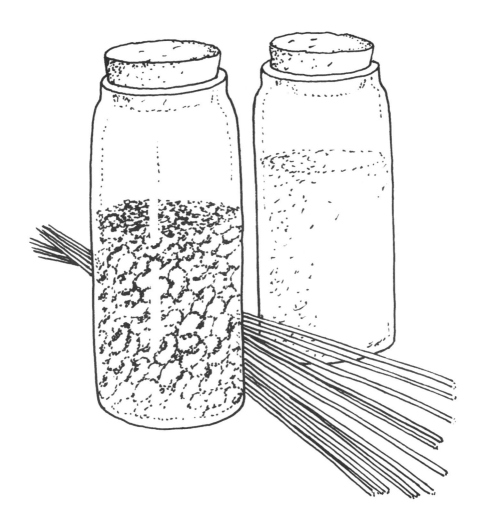

BAKED RICE

Exchanges: 1 Starch

Serving Size: ⅓ cup
Carbohydrate: 19 gm
Protein: 3 gm
Fat: 1 gm

Calories: 98
Fiber: 0 gm
Sodium: 473 mg
Cholesterol: 1 mg

INGREDIENTS:

1 cup long-grain rice, uncooked
Vegetable cooking spray
1 (10½-ounce) can beef
   consommé, undiluted

1 (10½-ounce) can onion soup
   in beef stock, undiluted

STEPS IN PREPARATION:

1. Place rice in a 1-quart casserole coated with cooking spray.
2. Pour consommé and soup over rice; stir well.
3. Cover and bake at 350° for 1 hour, stirring occasionally.

Yield: 9 servings

Increase the flavor of rice without adding a lot of
fat or calories by cooking it in chicken broth, beef
broth, or consommé. You can also use orange juice
or apple juice as the cooking liquid to add zest to
rice. Be sure to count the juice in your meal plan.

BAKED CHEESE AND RICE

Exchanges: 1 Starch, ½ Medium-Fat Meat

Serving Size: ⅓ cup
Carbohydrate: 19 gm
Protein: 6 gm
Fat: 3 gm

Calories: 130
Fiber: 0 gm
Sodium: 560 mg
Cholesterol: 9 mg

INGREDIENTS:

¾ cup skim milk
1 cup (4 ounces) shredded
  low-fat process American
  cheese
1 teaspoon reduced-calorie
  margarine
½ teaspoon Worcestershire
  sauce

¼ teaspoon salt
Dash of pepper
2 cups cooked long-grain rice
  (cooked without salt or fat)
Vegetable cooking spray
Dash of paprika

STEPS IN PREPARATION:

1. Combine milk and cheese in a small saucepan; cook over low heat, stirring constantly, until cheese melts.
2. Add margarine and next 3 ingredients; stir well. Add rice, and stir.
3. Spoon mixture into a 1-quart baking dish coated with cooking spray; sprinkle with paprika. Bake at 350° for 15 minutes or until lightly browned.

Yield: 7 servings

BLACK-EYED PEAS WITH RICE

Exchanges: 1 Starch

Serving Size: ⅓ cup	**Calories:** 92
Carbohydrate: 17 gm	**Fiber:** 5 gm
Protein: 5 gm	**Sodium:** 316 mg
Fat: 1 gm	**Cholesterol:** 0 mg

INGREDIENTS:

½ cup chopped onion
2 teaspoons reduced-calorie margarine, melted
⅔ cup cooked long-grain rice (cooked without salt or fat)
¼ teaspoon salt
¼ teaspoon pepper

1 (15-ounce) can black-eyed peas, drained
1 (14½-ounce) can stewed tomatoes, undrained
Vegetable cooking spray

STEPS IN PREPARATION:

1. Sauté onion in margarine in a nonstick skillet until tender.
2. Add rice and next 4 ingredients, stirring well.
3. Spoon mixture into a 1-quart casserole coated with cooking spray. Bake at 350° for 30 minutes or until thoroughly heated.

Yield: 9 servings

Legumes, such as black-eyed peas, chick-peas, lima beans, and kidney beans, are packed with complex carbohydrates, fiber, vitamins, minerals, and protein—more protein than any other edible plant food. Legumes have no cholesterol, are very low in fat and sodium, and are inexpensive.

HAM "FRIED" RICE

Exchanges: 1 Starch, 1 Medium-Fat Meat

Serving Size: ¾ cup
Carbohydrate: 19 gm
Protein: 9 gm
Fat: 4 gm

Calories: 150
Fiber: 1 gm
Sodium: 812 mg
Cholesterol: 18 mg

INGREDIENTS:

1 cup chopped celery
½ cup chopped onion
½ cup chopped green pepper
1 tablespoon reduced-calorie margarine, melted
1½ cups diced lean cooked ham

½ teaspoon salt
1 teaspoon curry powder
Dash of garlic powder
2 cups cooked long-grain rice (cooked without salt or fat)

STEPS IN PREPARATION:

1. Sauté celery, onion, and green pepper in margarine in a large nonstick skillet.
2. Add ham and next 3 ingredients, stirring well. Stir in rice. Cook over medium heat, stirring constantly, until thoroughly heated.

Yield: 7 servings

HOLIDAY RICE

Exchanges: 1 Starch

Serving Size: ½ cup
Carbohydrate: 19 gm
Protein: 2 gm
Fat: 1 gm

Calories: 99
Fiber: 1 gm
Sodium: 496 mg
Cholesterol: 0 mg

INGREDIENTS:

½ cup chopped onion
½ cup chopped celery
½ cup chopped green pepper
2 tablespoons reduced-calorie margarine, melted
2½ cups cooked long-grain rice (cooked without salt or fat)

1 cup cooked chopped broccoli
2 tablespoons chopped fresh parsley
1 teaspoon salt
Vegetable cooking spray
Fresh parsley sprigs (optional)

STEPS IN PREPARATION:

1. Sauté first 3 ingredients in margarine in a nonstick skillet.
2. Add rice, broccoli, chopped parsley, and salt; stir well.
3. Spoon mixture into a warm 5-cup ring mold coated with cooking spray, and invert onto a serving platter.
4. Garnish with parsley sprigs, if desired.

Yield: 9 servings

MEXICAN RICE

Exchanges: 1 Starch

Serving Size: ⅓ cup
Carbohydrate: 19 gm
Protein: 2 gm
Fat: 1 gm

Calories: 94
Fiber: 1 gm
Sodium: 485 mg
Cholesterol: 0 mg

INGREDIENTS:

⅔ cup chopped onion
1 tablespoon reduced-calorie margarine, melted
1 cup long-grain rice, uncooked
1 cup chopped green pepper

1 teaspoon salt
1 teaspoon chili powder
1 (8-ounce) can whole tomatoes, chopped
2 cups water

STEPS IN PREPARATION:

1. Sauté onion in margarine in a nonstick skillet until tender.
2. Stir in rice and next 4 ingredients; add water.
3. Bring to boil; reduce heat, cover, and simmer 20 minutes or until rice is tender and liquid is absorbed.

Yield: 10 servings

To cook the perfect pot of rice, remember that cooking times vary with brands and the amount of liquid recommended by each. Follow the package directions for each brand for best results. These directions usually indicate how to make rice firmer or softer to suit personal taste. You can interchange most kinds of rice in different recipes by making minor adjustments.

PARTY RICE

Exchanges: 1 Starch, 1 High-Fat Meat, 1 Fat

Serving Size: ½ cup	**Calories:** 234
Carbohyrate: 19 gm	**Fiber:** 2 gm
Protein: 8 gm	**Sodium:** 830 mg
Fat: 14 gm	**Cholesterol:** 42 mg

INGREDIENTS:

1 cup cooked long-grain rice (cooked without salt or fat)

1 cup diced fresh mushrooms

1 cup (4 ounces) shredded low-fat process American cheese

1 cup canned cream of mushroom soup, undiluted

½ cup pecans or almonds, chopped

1 egg, lightly beaten

1 (4-ounce) jar pimiento, drained and chopped

Vegetable cooking spray

Fresh parsley (optional)

STEPS IN PREPARATION:

1. Combine first 7 ingredients in a medium bowl. Spoon into a 1-quart baking dish coated with cooking spray.
2. Cover and bake at 350° for 30 minutes or until thoroughly heated.
3. Garnish with fresh parsley, if desired.

Yield: 6 servings

PARSLIED RICE

Exchanges: 1 Starch, 1 Medium-Fat Meat

Serving Size: ½ cup	**Calories:** 177
Carbohydrate: 17 gm	**Fiber:** 1 gm
Protein: 11 gm	**Sodium:** 642 mg
Fat: 7 gm	**Cholesterol:** 39 mg

INGREDIENTS:

2 green onions, chopped
½ clove garlic, minced
3 tablespoons reduced-calorie margarine, melted
2 cups cooked long-grain rice (cooked without salt or fat)
2 cups skim milk
2 cups (8 ounces) shredded low-fat process American cheese
1 cup chopped fresh parsley
½ teaspoon salt
1 egg, lightly beaten
Vegetable cooking spray

STEPS IN PREPARATION:

1. Sauté onions and garlic in margarine in a nonstick skillet until tender.
2. Combine onion mixture, rice, and next 5 ingredients, stirring well.
3. Spoon mixture into a 1½-quart casserole coated with cooking spray. Bake at 350° for 45 minutes or until thoroughly heated.

Yield: 8 servings

WILD RICE CASSEROLE

Exchanges: 1 Starch

Serving Size: ½ cup
Carbohydrate: 10 gm
Protein: 2 gm
Fat: 2 gm

Calories: 69
Fiber: 1 gm
Sodium: 374 mg
Cholesterol: trace

INGREDIENTS:

1 (10-ounce) package brown
   and wild rice mix
1 teaspoon salt
1 medium onion, minced
1 medium-size green pepper,
   chopped
2 tablespoons reduced-calorie
   margarine, melted

½ cup skim milk
½ (10¾-ounce) can cream of
   mushroom soup, undiluted
1 (4-ounce) jar whole pimiento,
   drained and minced
Vegetable cooking spray

STEPS IN PREPARATION:

1. Cook rice according to package directions, using 1 teaspoon salt.
   Set aside.
2. Sauté onion and green pepper in margarine in a nonstick skillet
   until tender.
3. Combine rice, onion mixture, milk, soup, and pimiento, stirring
   well. Spoon into a 1½-quart casserole coated with cooking spray.
   Bake at 350° for 30 minutes or until thoroughly heated.

Yield: 10 servings

VEGETABLE-RICE CASSEROLE

Exchanges: 2 Starch

Serving Size: ½ cup
Carbohydrate: 28 gm
Protein: 5 gm
Fat: 2 gm

Calories: 147
Fiber: 4 gm
Sodium: 582 mg
Cholesterol: trace

INGREDIENTS:

2 teaspoons vegetable oil
2 cups chopped cauliflower
2 cups chopped broccoli
1 cup chopped onion, divided
2 medium-size green peppers, cut into strips
2 cloves garlic, chopped
½ teaspoon dried thyme

1 tablespoon chicken-flavored bouillon granules
3 cups hot water
1½ cups brown rice, uncooked
3 tablespoons reduced-sodium soy sauce

STEPS IN PREPARATION:

1. Place oil in a large skillet; add cauliflower, broccoli, ½ cup onion, green pepper, and garlic. Sauté 5 minutes or until tender. Stir in thyme. Remove from heat, and set aside.
2. Dissolve bouillon granules in hot water in a 2-quart casserole. Stir in remaining ½ cup onion, rice, and soy sauce. Cover and bake at 350° for 20 minutes.
3. Remove casserole from oven, and stir in vegetable mixture. Cover and bake 10 to 15 minutes or until liquid is absorbed.

Yield: 10 servings

RED BEANS AND RICE

Exchanges: 1½ Starch

Serving Size: ½ cup
Carbohydrate: 20 gm
Protein: 6 gm
Fat: trace

Calories: 106
Fiber: 5 gm
Sodium: 304 mg
Cholesterol: trace

INGREDIENTS:

Vegetable cooking spray
½ cup finely chopped celery
¼ cup chopped green onions
¼ cup chopped green pepper
1 (16-ounce) can kidney
  beans, drained
1 teaspoon beef-flavored
  bouillon granules
1 cup boiling water

1 teaspoon garlic powder
1 teaspoon dried oregano
½ teaspoon ground white
  pepper
⅛ teaspoon ground red
  pepper
1 cup cooked long-grain rice
  (cooked without salt or fat)

STEPS IN PREPARATION:

1. Coat a medium nonstick skillet with cooking spray. Place over medium heat until hot. Add celery, green onions, and green pepper; sauté 5 minutes or until tender. Stir in beans.
2. Dissolve bouillon granules in boiling water. Add to vegetable mixture. Stir in garlic powder and next 3 ingredients; bring to a boil.
3. Add cooked rice to skillet, stirring well. Cover and remove from heat. Let stand 5 minutes.

Yield: 8 servings

BLACK BEANS AND RICE

Exchanges: 3 Starch

Serving Size: 1 cup
Carbohydrate: 48 gm
Protein: 12 gm
Fat: trace

Calories: 246
Fiber: 9 gm
Sodium: 240 mg
Cholesterol: 0 mg

INGREDIENTS:

- 1 (16-ounce) package dried black beans
- 1 medium-size green pepper, chopped
- ¼ cup chopped onion, divided
- 2½ quarts water, divided

- ½ teaspoon dried oregano
- ¼ teaspoon ground cumin
- 2 cloves garlic, minced
- 3 tablespoons vinegar
- 1 teaspoon salt
- 3 cups cooked long-grain rice

(cooked without salt or fat)

STEPS IN PREPARATION:

1. Sort and wash beans. Combine beans, green pepper, and 2 tablespoons onion in a large Dutch oven. Cover with 6 cups of water, and soak overnight.
2. Add remaining 4 cups water to Dutch oven; cover and bring to a boil. Reduce heat, and simmer 2½ hours or until beans are tender.
3. Combine remaining 2 tablespoons onion, oregano, cumin, and garlic in a small bowl; mash mixture, using a fork. Stir in vinegar.
4. Add vinegar mixture and salt to beans. Simmer, uncovered, an additional 20 minutes. Serve over ⅓-cup portions of cooked rice.

Yield: 9 servings

MACARONI AND CHEESE

Exchanges: 1 Starch, 1 Medium-Fat Meat

Serving Size: ½ cup
Carbohydrate: 22 gm
Protein: 8 gm
Fat: 4 gm

Calories: 160
Fiber: 1 gm
Sodium: 547 mg
Cholesterol: 9 mg

INGREDIENTS:

1½ tablespoons all-purpose
   flour
1½ cups skim milk, divided
1½ tablespoons reduced-
   calorie margarine
½ teaspoon salt
¾ cup (3 ounces) shredded
   low-fat process American
   cheese

2 cups cooked macaroni
   (cooked without salt or fat)
Vegetable cooking spray
¼ cup soft breadcrumbs

STEPS IN PREPARATION:

1. Combine flour and ¼ cup milk in a saucepan; stir until smooth.
   Add remaining 1¼ cups milk and margarine; stir well. Cook over
   medium heat, stirring constantly, until thickened and bubbly.
   Remove from heat, and add salt.
2. Add cheese, and cook over low heat, stirring constantly, until
   cheese melts. Remove from heat.
3. Alternate layers of macaroni and cheese sauce in a 1-quart
   casserole coated with cooking spray; top with breadcrumbs. Bake
   at 375° until mixture is bubbly and lightly browned.

Yield: 6 servings

FETTUCCINE ALFREDO

Exchanges: 2 Starch, 1 Fat

Serving Size: ½ cup
Carbohydrate: 29 gm
Protein: 7 gm
Fat: 4 gm

Calories: 187
Fiber: 2 gm
Sodium: 114 mg
Cholesterol: 39 mg

INGREDIENTS:

12 ounces fettuccine, uncooked
3 tablespoons reduced-calorie margarine
1 tablespoon all-purpose flour
½ cup skim milk
¼ cup grated Parmesan cheese

STEPS IN PREPARATION:

1. Cook fettuccine according to package directions, omitting salt and fat. Drain well; place in a large bowl, and keep warm.
2. Melt margarine in a medium saucepan over low heat; add flour. Cook, stirring constantly, 3 to 4 minutes or until smooth.
3. Add milk to flour mixture, and place over medium heat. Cook, stirring constantly, until mixture is thickened and bubbly.
4. Reduce heat to low, and stir in cheese. Cook, stirring constantly, until cheese melts and sauce is smooth.
5. Pour sauce over fettuccine, and toss gently to coat. Serve immediately.

Yield: 8 servings

FRESH BROCCOLI AND NOODLES

Exchanges: 1 Starch, ½ Fat

Serving Size: ½ cup	**Calories:** 89
Carbohydrate: 13 gm	**Fiber:** 4 gm
Protein: 4 gm	**Sodium:** 105 mg
Fat: 3 gm	**Cholesterol:** 9 mg

INGREDIENTS:

3 ounces medium egg noodles, uncooked
Vegetable cooking spray
3 cups broccoli flowerets
2 cups sliced fresh mushrooms
¼ cup chopped onion
¼ teaspoon garlic powder
¼ teaspoon coarsely ground black pepper
⅛ teaspoon salt
3 tablespoons reduced-calorie margarine

STEPS IN PREPARATION:

1. Cook noodles according to package directions, omitting salt and fat; drain and set aside.
2. Coat a wok or large nonstick skillet with cooking spray. Heat at medium-high (375°) for 2 minutes. Add broccoli, mushrooms, and onion; stir-fry 4 minutes or until broccoli is tender.
3. Add garlic powder, pepper, and salt to wok. Stir in noodles and margarine; cook over medium-high heat, stirring gently, until thoroughly heated.

Yield: 8 servings

PARSLIED NOODLES

Exchanges: 1 Starch, ½ Fat

Serving Size: ⅓ cup	**Calories:** 94
Carbohydrate: 13 gm	**Fiber:** 1 gm
Protein: 3 gm	**Sodium:** 164 mg
Fat: 3 gm	**Cholesterol:** 17 mg

INGREDIENTS:

6 ounces medium egg noodles, uncooked

¼ cup reduced-calorie margarine, melted

2 tablespoons chopped fresh parsley

Dash of garlic powder

2 tablespoons grated Parmesan cheese

STEPS IN PREPARATION:

1. Cook noodles according to package directions, omitting salt and fat; drain well. Pour margarine over noodles.
2. Add parsley and garlic powder; toss gently to coat. Sprinkle with cheese.

Yield: 9 servings

Dried pasta can be kept almost indefinitely if you store it in an airtight container in a cool, dry place. Fresh pasta is highly perishable and should be kept in an airtight container in the refrigerator and used within a week.

CREAMY LINGUINE

Exchanges: 1 Starch, ½ Fat

Serving Size: ½ cup	**Calories:** 100
Carbohydrate: 14 gm	**Fiber:** 1 gm
Protein: 5 gm	**Sodium:** 116 mg
Fat: 2 gm	**Cholesterol:** 42 mg

INGREDIENTS:

2 ounces thin egg noodles, uncooked

2 ounces spinach linguine, uncooked

3 tablespoons skim milk

1 egg, lightly beaten

¼ cup grated Parmesan cheese

1 tablespoon sliced pimiento

STEPS IN PREPARATION:

1. Cook pastas according to package directions, omitting salt and fat. Drain well; place in a large bowl, and keep warm.
2. Combine milk and egg in a small saucepan; cook over low heat 2 minutes, stirring frequently with a wire whisk. Stir in cheese and pimiento. Remove from heat.
3. Pour cheese mixture over pasta, and toss gently to coat. Serve immediately.

Yield: 6 servings

VEGETABLES AND PASTA IN CHEESE SAUCE

Exchanges: 1 Starch

Serving Size: ½ cup
Carbohydrate: 10 gm
Protein: 4 gm
Fat: 1 gm

Calories: 70
Fiber: 2 gm
Sodium: 177 mg
Cholesterol: 4 mg

INGREDIENTS:

2 cups cauliflower flowerets
2 cups diagonally sliced carrot
¼ cup minced onion
2 teaspoons reduced-calorie margarine, melted
1 tablespoon all-purpose flour
1 cup skim milk

½ cup (2 ounces) shredded reduced-fat Cheddar cheese
¼ teaspoon Worcestershire sauce
⅛ teaspoon salt
⅛ teaspoon pepper
½ cup cooked corkscrew or shell macaroni (cooked without salt or fat)

STEPS IN PREPARATION:

1. Combine cauliflower and carrot in a medium saucepan; add water to cover. Cover and bring to a boil. Reduce heat, and simmer 15 minutes or until vegetables are tender. Drain well; set aside, and keep warm.
2. Sauté onion in margarine in saucepan 2 minutes or until tender. Add flour, stirring well; cook, stirring constantly, 1 minute. Gradually add milk; cook over medium heat, stirring constantly, until mixture is thickened and bubbly.
3. Reduce heat to low, and add cheese and next 3 ingredients. Cook, stirring constantly, until cheese melts.
4. Add vegetables and pasta to cheese sauce in saucepan, stirring gently to coat vegetables and pasta. Cook over low heat until mixture is thoroughly heated, stirring gently.

Yield: 9 servings

VERMICELLI WITH TOMATO SAUCE

Exchanges: 1 Starch, 1½ Vegetable

Serving Size: 1 cup
Carbohydrate: 25 gm
Protein: 4 gm
Fat: 1 gm

Calories: 123
Fiber: 2 gm
Sodium: 286 mg
Cholesterol: 0 mg

INGREDIENTS:

½ cup chopped onion
1 teaspoon reduced-calorie margarine, melted
3 cups peeled, chopped tomato
1 teaspoon paprika

½ teaspoon salt
½ teaspoon dried basil
½ teaspoon dried oregano
⅛ teaspoon pepper
3 cups cooked vermicelli (cooked without salt or fat)

STEPS IN PREPARATION:

1. Sauté onion in margarine in a nonstick skillet.
2. Add tomato and next 5 ingredients; cover and simmer 5 minutes, stirring occasionally.
3. Remove from heat, and spoon over ½-cup portions of pasta.

Yield: 6 servings

Vermicelli is very thin pasta. Substitute thin spaghetti or angel hair pasta if vermicelli is not available.

LIMA BEANS DELUXE

Exchanges: 1 Starch, 1 Lean Meat

Serving Size: ½ cup
Carbohydrate: 16 gm
Protein: 7 gm
Fat: 3 gm

Calories: 115
Fiber: 3 gm
Sodium: 450 mg
Cholesterol: 6 mg

INGREDIENTS:

1 (10-ounce) package frozen
  lima beans
1 tablespoon reduced-calorie
  margarine
1 tablespoon all-purpose
  flour
1 cup skim milk
½ teaspoon salt

⅛ teaspoon pepper
½ cup (2 ounces) shredded
  reduced-fat Cheddar cheese
2 tablespoons reduced-calorie
  ketchup
2 (4-ounce) jars diced
  pimiento, drained
Vegetable cooking spray

STEPS IN PREPARATION:

1. Cook beans according to package directions, omitting salt and fat. Drain and set aside.
2. Melt margarine in a medium saucepan over low heat; add flour, stirring until smooth. Cook, stirring constantly, 1 minute. Gradually add milk; cook over medium heat, stirring constantly, until thickened and bubbly. Stir in salt and pepper. Remove from heat.
3. Add beans, cheese, ketchup, and pimiento to sauce; stir well. Spoon into a 1½-quart casserole coated with cooking spray. Bake at 375° for 30 minutes or until thoroughly heated.

Yield: 6 servings

ROASTED CORN ON THE COB

Exchanges: 1 Starch, ½ Fat

Serving Size: ½ ear	**Calories:** 83
Carbohydrate: 16 gm	**Fiber:** 2 gm
Protein: 2 gm	**Sodium:** 123 mg
Fat: 3 gm	**Cholesterol:** 0 mg

INGREDIENTS:

2 (8-inch) ears fresh corn
4 teaspoons reduced-calorie
    margarine

Dash of salt
Dash of pepper

STEPS IN PREPARATION:

1. Turn back corn husks, and remove silk.
2. Spread margarine evenly on corn; sprinkle with salt and pepper.
3. Pull husks back up, tying tightly.
4. Place corn on grill rack. Grill over hot coals (400° to 500°),
   uncovered, for 30 minutes, turning frequently.
5. To serve, remove ears from husks, and cut each in half.

Yield: 4 servings

SKILLET CORN

Exchanges: 1 Starch

Serving Size: ⅓ cup
Carbohydrate: 12 gm
Protein: 2 gm
Fat: 1 gm

Calories: 58
Fiber: 2 gm
Sodium: 391 mg
Cholesterol: 0 mg

INGREDIENTS:

10 ears fresh corn (about 2
    cups cut corn)
½ cup skim milk
1 teaspoon salt

⅛ teaspoon pepper
1 tablespoon reduced-calorie
    margarine

STEPS IN PREPARATION:

1. Shuck corn, and remove silk from ears. Cut kernels from cobs.
   Scrape cobs gently with back of knife to get juice.
2. Add milk, salt, and pepper to corn, and stir.
3. Melt margarine in a heavy skillet. Pour corn mixture into skillet.
   Simmer until tender, stirring frequently.

Yield: 6 servings

Use fresh corn, green beans, and peas as soon as
possible because their sweet taste diminishes with
the length of storage as their sugar content turns
to starch. Store these vegetables, unwashed, in
plastic bags in the refrigerator for short periods of
time only.

MEXICAN CORN

Exchanges: 1 Starch

Serving Size: ⅓ cup	**Calories:** 63
Carbohydrate: 12 gm	**Fiber:** 2 gm
Protein: 2 gm	**Sodium:** 349 mg
Fat: 2 gm	**Cholesterol:** 0 mg

INGREDIENTS:

2 cups canned whole kernel corn, drained
½ cup diced onion
¼ cup chopped green pepper
¼ cup chopped sweet red pepper

2 tablespoons reduced-calorie margarine, melted
1 teaspoon salt
¼ teaspoon dried oregano
¼ teaspoon ground allspice
1 cup peeled, diced tomato

STEPS IN PREPARATION:

1. Combine first 8 ingredients in a large nonstick skillet. Cover and cook over medium heat 7 minutes, stirring occasionally.
2. Add tomato; cook, uncovered, 2 minutes or until thoroughly heated.

Yield: 7 servings

CORN CUSTARD

Exchanges: 1 Starch, 1 Fat

Serving Size: ⅓ cup
Carbohydrate: 13 gm
Protein: 4 gm
Fat: 4 gm

Calories: 98
Fiber: 2 gm
Sodium: 343 mg
Cholesterol: 64 mg

INGREDIENTS:

1 (16-ounce) can cream-style
  corn
1 tablespoon chopped parsley

½ teaspoon onion salt
2 eggs, lightly beaten
Vegetable cooking spray

STEPS IN PREPARATION:

1. Combine first 4 ingredients in a medium bowl, stirring well.
2. Spoon mixture into a 1-quart casserole coated with cooking spray. Place casserole in a pan of warm water. Bake at 325° for 1¼ hours or until set. Serve warm.

Yield: 6 servings

If you want to reduce sodium, use canned no-salt-added cream-style corn instead of the regular product in this recipe and others.

CORN PUDDING

Exchanges: 1 Starch

Serving Size: ¼ cup
Carbohydrate: 10 gm
Protein: 4 gm
Fat: 2 gm

Calories: 62
Fiber: 1 gm
Sodium: 295 mg
Cholesterol: 47 mg

INGREDIENTS:

2 cups canned whole kernel
  corn, drained
1 cup skim milk
Sugar substitute to equal 1
  teaspoon sugar*
½ teaspoon salt

¼ teaspoon pepper
⅛ teaspoon ground allspice
2 eggs, well beaten
Vegetable cooking spray

STEPS IN PREPARATION:

1. Combine first 7 ingredients in a medium bowl, stirring well.
2. Spoon mixture into a 1-quart casserole coated with cooking spray. Bake at 350° for 60 to 70 minutes or until a knife inserted into center of pudding comes out clean. Serve warm.

Yield: 8 servings

*See the sugar substitution chart on page 354.

HASH BROWN POTATOES

Exchanges: 1 Starch

Serving Size: ½ cup	**Calories:** 67
Carbohydrate: 16 gm	**Fiber:** 1 gm
Protein: 1 gm	**Sodium:** 270 mg
Fat: trace	**Cholesterol:** 0 mg

INGREDIENTS:

Vegetable cooking spray
2 cups diced potato
½ teaspoon salt

¼ teaspoon pepper
¼ cup green onions (optional)

STEPS IN PREPARATION:

1. Coat a nonstick skillet with cooking spray. Place potato, salt, and pepper in skillet; cook over medium-high heat, stirring constantly, 2 minutes.
2. Reduce heat, and add onions, if desired; cook 30 minutes or until potato is tender, stirring occasionally.

Yield: 4 servings

Always store potatoes and onions in a well-ventilated cool, dark place to prevent them from sprouting. But don't store potatoes and onions together—the onions will absorb moisture from the potatoes, causing the onions to spoil faster.

HERBED NEW POTATOES

Exhanges: 1 Starch

Serving Size: 1 potato	**Calories:** 100
Carbohydrate: 22 gm	**Fiber:** 2 gm
Protein: 2 gm	**Sodium:** 112 mg
Fat: 1 gm	**Cholesterol:** 0 mg

INGREDIENTS:

6 small new potatoes
1 tablespoon minced fresh
   parsley
2 teaspoons reduced-calorie
   margarine

¼ teaspoon salt
Dash of pepper

STEPS IN PREPARATION:

1. Cook potatoes, covered, in boiling water to cover 20 minutes or until tender. Drain and peel potatoes.
2. Combine parsley and remaining ingredients; add to potatoes, tossing to coat.

Yield: 6 servings

POTATO CASSEROLE

Exchanges: 1 Starch, ½ Fat

Serving Size: ½ cup
Carbohydrate: 16 gm
Protein: 2 gm
Fat: 3 gm

Calories: 94
Fiber: 1 gm
Sodium: 445 mg
Cholesterol: 0 mg

INGREDIENTS:

4 medium baking potatoes,
  peeled and sliced
2 tablespoons chopped green
  pepper
2 tablespoons minced onion

½ teaspoon salt
⅛ teaspoon pepper
1 (10¾-ounce) can cream of
  mushroom soup, undiluted
Vegetable cooking spray

STEPS IN PREPARATION:

1. Combine first 6 ingredients in a medium bowl.
2. Spoon mixture into a 1-quart casserole coated with cooking spray.
   Bake at 350° for 1 to 1½ hours or until potato is tender.

Yield: 8 servings

Potatoes are practically fat-free and are a good
source of vitamins, minerals, and fiber. It's addi-
tions such as butter and sour cream that can make
potatoes fattening. Instead, try topping your potato
with nonfat yogurt or sour cream, low-fat Ranch
salad dressing, low-fat shredded cheese, vegetables, or salsa.

TWICE-BAKED POTATOES

Exchanges: 1 Starch

Serving Size: ½ potato
Carbohydrate: 14 gm
Protein: 3 gm
Fat: trace

Calories: 74
Fiber: 1 gm
Sodium: 75 mg
Cholesterol: 2 mg

INGREDIENTS:

4 small baking potatoes
½ cup skim milk
½ cup plain nonfat
   yogurt

¼ cup (1 ounce) shredded
   low-fat process American
   cheese
½ teaspoon paprika

STEPS IN PREPARATION:

1. Wash potatoes, and pat dry; prick each potato several times with a fork. Arrange potatoes end to end and 1 inch apart in a circle on paper towels in microwave oven. Microwave at HIGH 12 minutes, turning and rearranging potatoes after 6 minutes. Let potatoes stand 5 minutes.
2. Cut potatoes in half lengthwise. Scoop out pulp, leaving shells intact. Set shells aside.
3. Mash pulp in a large bowl, using a fork or potato masher. Add milk and yogurt; beat at low speed of an electric mixer until smooth and well blended. Spoon potato mixture into shells, and place on a microwave-safe serving platter.
4. Top stuffed potatoes evenly with cheese, and sprinkle with paprika. Microwave at HIGH 30 seconds or until cheese melts. Serve immediately.

Yield: 8 servings

SCALLOPED POTATOES

Exchanges: 1 Starch

Serving Size: ½ cup	**Calories:** 82
Carbohydrate: 17 gm	**Fiber:** 1 gm
Protein: 3 gm	**Sodium:** 144 mg
Fat: 1 gm	**Cholesterol:** trace

INGREDIENTS:

1 clove garlic, minced
1 tablespoon reduced-calorie margarine, melted
1 tablespoon cornstarch
½ teaspoon salt
⅛ teaspoon pepper
1½ cups skim milk

1½ pounds round red potatoes, peeled and thinly sliced
¼ cup chopped onion
¼ cup chopped fresh parsley
Vegetable cooking spray

STEPS IN PREPARATION:

1. Sauté garlic in margarine in a small saucepan until tender. Stir in cornstarch, salt, and pepper.
2. Add milk, stirring well. Cook over medium heat, stirring constantly, 2 minutes or until mixture is thickened and bubbly. Remove sauce from heat, and set aside.
3. Arrange half each of potato, onion, and parsley in a 2-quart casserole coated with cooking spray. Top with half of sauce. Repeat layers with remaining potato, onion, parsley, and sauce.
4. Cover and bake at 350° for 45 minutes, stirring once. Uncover and bake an additional 30 minutes or until potato is tender.

Yield: 10 servings

POTATO-CHEESE CASSEROLE

Exchanges: 1 Starch, ½ Fat

Serving Size: ½ cup	**Calories:** 103
Carbohydrate: 18 gm	**Fiber:** 1 gm
Protein: 4 gm	**Sodium:** 215 mg
Fat: 2 gm	**Cholesterol:** 27 mg

INGREDIENTS:

3 cups cooked, mashed potato (cooked without salt or fat)
1 egg, separated
½ cup (2 ounces) shredded low-fat process American cheese
1 tablespoon finely chopped green onions
½ teaspoon celery salt
½ small green pepper, finely chopped
1 egg white
Vegetable cooking spray
½ teaspoon paprika

STEPS IN PREPARATION:

1. Combine mashed potato and egg yolk, stirring until well blended. Stir in cheese, green onions, celery salt, and green pepper.
2. Beat 2 egg whites (at room temperature) at high speed of an electric mixer until soft peaks form. Gently fold egg whites into potato mixture.
3. Spoon mixture into a 1½-quart casserole coated with cooking spray. Sprinkle paprika evenly over top of casserole. Bake at 375° for 25 to 30 minutes or until thoroughly heated.

Yield: 8 servings

SWEET POTATO CASSEROLE

Exchanges: 1½ Starch, ½ Fat

Serving Size: ⅓ cup
Carbohydrate: 24 gm
Protein: 3 gm
Fat: 3 gm

Calories: 132
Fiber: 1 gm
Sodium: 96 mg
Cholesterol: 31 mg

INGREDIENTS:

1 (18-ounce) can sweet
  potatoes, drained
1 cup granulated brown
  sugar substitute, divided
¼ cup skim milk
1 tablespoon reduced-calorie
  margarine, melted

1 teaspoon vanilla extract
1 egg
Vegetable cooking spray
1 tablespoon all-purpose flour
1 tablespoon reduced-calorie
  margarine

STEPS IN PREPARATION:

1. Combine sweet potato, ¾ cup brown sugar substitute, and next 4
   ingredients, stirring until well blended. Spoon mixture into a
   shallow baking dish coated with cooking spray.
2. Combine flour and remaining ¼ cup brown sugar substitute; cut
   in 1 tablespoon margarine until mixture is crumbly.
3. Sprinkle flour mixture over potatoes, and bake at 350° for 35
   minutes or until thoroughly heated.

Yield: 6 servings

SPICED SWEET POTATOES

Exchanges: 1 Starch, ½ Fat

Serving Size: ¼ cup	**Calories:** 86
Carbohydrate: 14 gm	**Fiber:** 2 gm
Protein: 1 gm	**Sodium:** 182 mg
Fat: 3 gm	**Cholesterol:** 0 mg

INGREDIENTS:

2 cups cooked or canned
  sliced sweet potatoes
Vegetable cooking spray
3 tablespoons granulated
  brown sugar substitute

¼ teaspoon salt
¼ teaspoon ground cinnamon
¼ teaspoon ground nutmeg
3 tablespoons reduced-calorie
  margarine

STEPS IN PREPARATION:

1. Arrange sweet potato in a 1½-quart casserole coated with cooking spray.
2. Combine sugar substitute, salt, cinnamon, and nutmeg; sprinkle over sweet potatoes. Dot with margarine. Bake at 350° for 10 to 15 minutes or until thoroughly heated.

Yield: 6 servings

Choose sweet potatoes that are firm, plump, blemish-free, and of uniform size. Store them in a cool, dry, well-ventilated place for up to two months. (Don't refrigerate them.) For longer storage, cook, mash, and then freeze sweet potatoes.

Vegetables

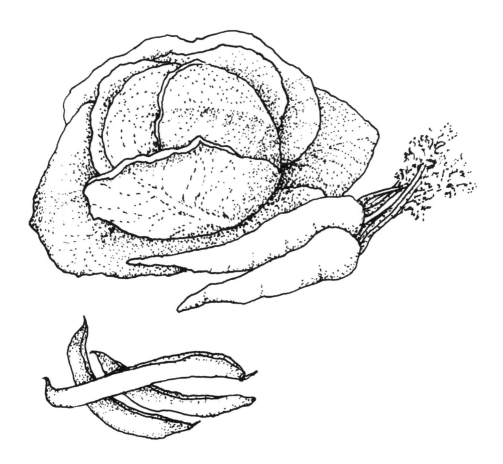

ASPARAGUS WITH HOT BACON DRESSING

Exchanges: 1 Vegetable, ½ Fat

Serving Size: ½ cup
Carbohydrate: 8 gm
Protein: 4 gm
Fat: 2 gm

Calories: 58
Fiber: 3 gm
Sodium: 453 mg
Cholesterol: 3 mg

INGREDIENTS:

2 slices bacon, finely diced
½ medium onion, finely chopped
¼ cup vinegar
¼ cup water

Sugar substitute to equal 2 teaspoons sugar*
1 (14½-ounce) can asparagus, heated and drained

STEPS IN PREPARATION:

1. Brown bacon in a skillet until crisp. Add onion, and cook until tender; drain well.
2. Add vinegar and water; bring to a boil.
3. Remove from heat, and stir in sugar substitute. Pour dressing over asparagus, and serve warm.

Yield: 4 servings

*See the sugar substitution chart on page 354.

ASPARAGUS WITH LEMON SAUCE

Exchanges: 1 Vegetable, ½ Fat

Serving Size: ½ cup
Carbohydrate: 7 gm
Protein: 1 gm
Fat: 2 gm

Calories: 49
Fiber: 1 gm
Sodium: 37 mg
Cholesterol: 31 mg

INGREDIENTS:

1 (10-ounce) package frozen asparagus spears
Sugar substitute to equal ½ cup sugar*
½ teaspoon cornstarch
1 egg

1 tablespoon reduced-calorie margarine
¼ cup lemon juice
2 teaspoons grated lemon rind

STEPS IN PREPARATION:

1. Cook asparagus according to package directions, omitting salt and fat; drain well. Transfer cooked asparagus to a serving dish, and keep warm.
2. Combine sugar substitute, cornstarch, and egg, stirring to blend. Melt margarine over low heat in a small skillet; add egg mixture. Cook over medium heat until mixture thickens.
3. Stir in lemon juice, and cook over medium heat until thickened and bubbly. Pour over asparagus, and sprinkle with lemon rind. Serve immediately.

Yield: 6 servings

*See the sugar substitution chart on page 354.

ASPARAGUS CASSEROLE

Exchanges: 1 Vegetable, ½ Fat

Serving Size: ½ cup	**Calories:** 55
Carbohydrate: 5 gm	**Fiber:** trace
Protein: 3 gm	**Sodium:** 435 mg
Fat: 2 gm	**Cholesterol:** 3 mg

INGREDIENTS:

1 (10-ounce) package frozen asparagus spears
½ cup skim milk
½ (10¾-ounce) can cream of mushroom soup, undiluted

1 (8-ounce) can sliced water chestnuts, drained
½ cup (2 ounces) shredded reduced-fat Cheddar cheese
Vegetable cooking spray

STEPS IN PREPARATION:

1. Cook asparagus according to package directions, omitting salt and fat; drain and set aside.
2. Combine milk and soup, stirring until blended. Layer half each of asparagus, soup mixture, water chestnuts, and cheese in a 1½-quart casserole coated with cooking spray.
3. Repeat layers with remaining asparagus, soup mixture, water chestnuts, and cheese. Bake at 325° for 20 minutes or until thoroughly heated.

Yield: 8 servings

PICKLED BEETS

Exchanges: 1 Vegetable

Serving Size: ½ cup	**Calories:** 32
Carbohydrate: 8 gm	**Fiber:** 2 gm
Protein: 1 gm	**Sodium:** 69 mg
Fat: trace	**Cholesterol:** 0 mg

INGREDIENTS:

1¾ cups canned sliced beets,
   drained
½ cup vinegar
Sugar substitute to equal 3
   tablespoons sugar*

6 whole cloves
1 slice lemon
1 small onion, thinly sliced

STEPS IN PREPARATION:

1. Place beets in a shallow dish; add vinegar and next 3 ingredients.
2. Separate onion slices into rings, and add to beets.
3. Cover and chill at least 4 hours.

Yield: 6 servings

*See the sugar substitution chart on page 354.

BROCCOLI CASSEROLE

Exchanges: 3 Vegetable, 1 Fat

Serving Size: 1 cup
Carbohydrate: 15 gm
Protein: 6 gm
Fat: 5 gm

Calories: 123
Fiber: 3 gm
Sodium: 681 mg
Cholesterol: 7 mg

INGREDIENTS:

1 pound fresh broccoli
1 cup water
½ teaspoon salt
¼ cup chopped onion
¼ cup chopped celery
¼ pound fresh mushrooms, sliced
2 teaspoons reduced-calorie margarine, melted
1 (8-ounce) can sliced water chestnuts, drained

½ cup (2 ounces) shredded low-fat process American cheese, divided
½ cup skim milk
½ (10¾-ounce) can cream of mushroom soup, undiluted
⅛ teaspoon garlic powder
⅛ teaspoon pepper
Vegetable cooking spray

STEPS IN PREPARATION:

1. Trim off large leaves of broccoli; remove tough ends of lower stalks. Wash thoroughly; cut into 1-inch pieces.
2. Bring water to a boil in a large saucepan; add broccoli and salt. Cover, reduce heat, and simmer 5 minutes or until tender. Drain and set aside.
3. Sauté onion, celery, and mushrooms in margarine in saucepan until tender. Combine broccoli, sautéed vegetables, and water chestnuts in a large bowl; set aside.
4. Combine ¼ cup cheese, milk, and soup in saucepan; cook over low heat, stirring constantly, until cheese melts. Stir in garlic powder and pepper. Pour over broccoli mixture, tossing to coat.
5. Spoon mixture into a 2-quart casserole coated with cooking spray. Bake at 350° for 25 minutes; sprinkle with remaining ¼ cup cheese. Bake an additional 5 minutes or until cheese melts.

Yield: 5 servings

CHINESE BROCCOLI

Exchanges: 2 Vegetable

Serving Size: ½ cup	**Calories:** 51
Carbohydrate: 8 gm	**Fiber:** 4 gm
Protein: 4 gm	**Sodium:** 177 mg
Fat: 1 gm	**Cholesterol:** 0 mg

INGREDIENTS:

1 pound fresh broccoli
Vegetable cooking spray
1 tablespoon reduced-sodium soy sauce
1 tablespoon sesame seeds, toasted
1 sweet red pepper, sliced

STEPS IN PREPARATION:

1. Trim off large leaves of broccoli; remove tough ends of lower stalks. Wash thoroughly; separate into spears, and cut into ¼-inch diagonal slices.
2. Arrange broccoli in a vegetable steamer over boiling water. Cover and steam 3 to 5 minutes or until crisp-tender.
3. Coat a large nonstick skillet with cooking spray. Add soy sauce, and place over medium heat until hot. Add broccoli; cook, stirring constantly, 1 to 2 minutes or until tender.
4. Transfer broccoli to a serving dish. Sprinkle with sesame seeds, and garnish with pepper slices.

Yield: 4 servings

Broccoli is one of the best nutrition bets in the produce section. A medium-size stalk provides 100 percent of the Recommended Daily Allowance for vitamin C. Broccoli is also rich in vitamin A, high in fiber, and low in calories.

BROCCOLI AND RICE CASSEROLE

Exchanges: 1 Starch, 1 Medium-Fat Meat, 1 Vegetable

Serving Size: ¾ cup	**Calories:** 188
Carbohydrate: 24 gm	**Fiber:** 2 gm
Protein: 9 gm	**Sodium:** 996 mg
Fat: 6 gm	**Cholesterol:** 14 mg

INGREDIENTS:

1 (10-ounce) package frozen chopped broccoli
½ cup chopped onion
½ cup chopped celery
1 teaspoon reduced-calorie margarine, melted
1 cup (4 ounces) grated reduced-fat Cheddar cheese
1 (10¾-ounce) can cream of chicken soup, undiluted
1½ cups cooked long-grain rice (cooked without salt or fat)
¼ teaspoon salt
¼ teaspoon hot sauce
⅛ teaspoon pepper
Vegetable cooking spray
1 tablespoon soft breadcrumbs

STEPS IN PREPARATION:

1. Cook broccoli according to package directions, omitting salt and fat; drain well.
2. Sauté onion and celery in margarine in a nonstick skillet until tender.
3. Combine broccoli, cheese, and soup; add to onion mixture. Stir in rice and next 3 ingredients.
4. Spoon mixture into a 1½-quart casserole coated with cooking spray; top with breadcrumbs. Bake at 350° for 45 minutes or until thoroughly heated.

Yield: 6 servings

GREEN BEAN CASSEROLE

Exchanges: ½ Medium-Fat Meat, 1 Vegetable

Serving Size: ½ cup
Carbohydrate: 5 gm
Protein: 4 gm
Fat: 2 gm

Calories: 54
Fiber: 2 gm
Sodium: 365 mg
Cholesterol: 72 mg

INGREDIENTS:

1 (10-ounce) package frozen chopped spinach, thawed
1 (9-ounce) package frozen green beans, thawed
½ cup chopped onion
¼ cup water
1 teaspoon salt
1 teaspoon dried basil
⅛ teaspoon garlic powder
⅛ teaspoon ground nutmeg
⅛ teaspoon pepper
3 eggs, lightly beaten
Vegetable cooking spray
¼ cup (1 ounce) shredded low-fat process American cheese
1 teaspoon paprika

STEPS IN PREPARATION:

1. Drain spinach and green beans well. Combine spinach, beans, onion, and next 6 ingredients in a medium saucepan. Cover and simmer 10 minutes, stirring occasionally. Remove from heat.
2. Gradually stir vegetable mixture into beaten eggs; stir well.
3. Spoon mixture into a 1-quart casserole coated with cooking spray. Bake, uncovered, at 350° for 20 minutes or until set.
4. Sprinkle with cheese and paprika; bake 2 to 3 minutes or until cheese melts.

Yield: 8 servings

SPANISH GREEN BEANS

Exchanges: 1 Vegetable, ½ Fat

Serving Size: ½ cup	**Calories:** 55
Carbohydrate: 10 gm	**Fiber:** 3 gm
Protein: 2 gm	**Sodium:** 449 mg
Fat: 2 gm	**Cholesterol:** 0 mg

INGREDIENTS:

3¾ cups fresh green beans
1 onion, chopped
2 tablespoons reduced-calorie margarine, melted
1½ teaspoons salt

½ teaspoon garlic powder
¼ teaspoon black pepper
5 medium tomatoes, diced
2 medium-size green peppers, chopped

STEPS IN PREPARATION:

1. Wash beans; trim ends, and remove strings. Cut beans into 1½-inch pieces.
2. Sauté onion in margarine in a nonstick skillet until tender.
3. Add beans, salt, garlic powder, and black pepper. Cover and cook over low heat 10 minutes, stirring frequently.
4. Stir in tomato and green pepper; cover and simmer 25 to 30 minutes or until beans are tender.

Yield: 8 servings

MARINATED GREEN BEANS AND ONIONS

Exchanges: 1 Vegetable

Serving Size: ½ cup
Carbohydrate: 5 gm
Protein: 2 gm
Fat: 1 gm

Calories: 32
Fiber: 3 gm
Sodium: 998 mg
Cholesterol: 8 mg

INGREDIENTS:

2 cups canned green beans, drained
1 cup commercial no-oil Italian salad dressing

¼ teaspoon salt
⅛ teaspoon pepper
1 small onion, sliced

STEPS IN PREPARATION:

1. Combine all ingredients in a large bowl, and stir well. Cover and chill at least 8 hours.
2. Serve warm or chilled.

Yield: 4 servings

Use canned no-salt-added green beans in this recipe and others to reduce the sodium content.

COPPER PENNIES

Exchanges: 1 Starch, ½ Fat

Serving Size: ¾ cup
Carbohydrate: 20 gm
Protein: 3 gm
Fat: 3 gm

Calories: 111
Fiber: 5 gm
Sodium: 462 mg
Cholesterol: 1 mg

INGREDIENTS:

3½ cups sliced carrot
2 medium onions, sliced
2 medium-size green peppers, sliced
½ cup skim milk
½ cup commercial no-oil Italian dressing

1 tablespoon prepared mustard
1 tablespoon Worcestershire sauce
½ (10¾-ounce) can tomato soup, undiluted

STEPS IN PREPARATION:

1. Cook carrot in boiling water to cover in a medium saucepan until tender; drain and cool. Add onion and green pepper.
2. Combine milk and remaining ingredients; pour over carrot mixture.
3. Cover and chill.

Yield: 6 servings

The darker the orange color of carrots, the more vitamin A they contain.

CARROTS VICHY

Exchanges: 2 Vegetable

Serving Size: ½ cup	**Calories:** 51
Carbohydrate: 10 gm	**Fiber:** 2 gm
Protein: 7 gm	**Sodium:** 432 mg
Fat: 1 gm	**Cholesterol:** 0 mg

INGREDIENTS:

1 tablespoon reduced-calorie margarine
3 cups sliced carrot
¾ cup water
1 teaspoon salt
¼ teaspoon ground nutmeg
⅛ teaspoon pepper
¼ cup chopped fresh parsley
1 tablespoon lemon juice
Sugar substitute to equal 2 teaspoons sugar*

STEPS IN PREPARATION:

1. Place margarine in a saucepan. Add carrot and next 4 ingredients.
2. Bring to a boil; reduce heat, cover, and simmer 8 to 10 minutes or until crisp-tender.
3. Stir in parsley, lemon juice, and sugar substitute. Serve warm.

Yield: 6 servings

*See the sugar substitution chart on page 354.

EGGPLANT CREOLE

Exchanges: ½ Starch

Serving Size: ½ cup	**Calories:** 36
Carbohydrate: 9 gm	**Fiber:** 2 gm
Protein: 1 gm	**Sodium:** 410 mg
Fat: trace	**Cholesterol:** 0 mg

INGREDIENTS:

1 small onion, chopped
1 small green pepper, chopped
1 (8-ounce) can tomato sauce
1 clove garlic, minced
½ teaspoon salt
¼ teaspoon oregano
¼ teaspoon hot sauce
⅛ teaspoon pepper
1 small eggplant, peeled and diced

STEPS IN PREPARATION:

1. Combine first 8 ingredients in a nonstick skillet. Cover and cook over low heat 10 minutes.
2. Add eggplant; cover and cook 20 minutes or until eggplant is tender, stirring occasionally.

Yield: 6 servings

Eggplant flesh darkens rapidly when cut, so don't peel it until just before cooking. Rub cut surfaces with lemon or lime juice to prevent darkening.

COMPANY CAULIFLOWER CASSEROLE

Exchanges: 1 Vegetable

Serving Size: ½ cup
Carbohydrate: 3 gm
Protein: 2 gm
Fat: 1 gm

Calories: 22
Fiber: trace
Sodium: 88 mg
Cholesterol: 1 mg

INGREDIENTS:

1 medium cauliflower, cut into flowerets
Vegetable cooking spray
½ teaspoon salt
⅛ teaspoon pepper
½ cup plain low-fat yogurt

2 tablespoons (½ ounce) shredded reduced-fat Cheddar cheese
1 teaspoon sesame seeds, toasted

STEPS IN PREPARATION:

1. Arrange cauliflower in a vegetable steamer over boiling water. Cover and steam 8 minutes or until tender.
2. Place half of cauliflower in a 1-quart casserole coated with cooking spray; sprinkle with salt and pepper. Top with half each of yogurt and cheese.
3. Repeat layers with remaining cauliflower, yogurt, and cheese. Sprinkle with sesame seeds, and bake at 350° for 20 minutes or until thoroughly heated.

Yield: 10 servings

SPINACH-CHEESE CASSEROLE

Exchanges: 1 Lean Meat, 1 Vegetable

Serving Size: ½ cup	**Calories:** 81
Carbohydrate: 6 gm	**Fiber:** 1 gm
Protein: 9 gm	**Sodium:** 318 mg
Fat: 3 gm	**Cholesterol:** 7 mg

INGREDIENTS:

1 (10-ounce) package frozen chopped spinach
1 medium onion, chopped
2 teaspoons reduced-calorie margarine, melted
1 cup 1% low-fat cottage cheese

¼ cup (1 ounce) shredded low-fat process American cheese, divided
⅛ teaspoon ground nutmeg
Dash of pepper
Vegetable cooking spray

STEPS IN PREPARATION:

1. Cook spinach according to package directions, omitting salt; drain well.
2. Sauté onion in margarine in a medium nonstick skillet until tender. Add spinach, cottage cheese, 2 tablespoons shredded cheese, nutmeg, and pepper; stir well.
3. Spoon into a 1-quart casserole coated wih cooking spray. Sprinkle with remaining 2 tablespoons shredded cheese. Bake at 350° for 25 to 30 minutes or until set.

Yield: 5 servings

OKRA CREOLE

Exchanges: 1 Vegetable

Serving Size: 1/3 cup	**Calories:** 36
Carbohydrate: 8 gm	**Fiber:** 2 gm
Protein: 1 gm	**Sodium:** 228 mg
Fat: trace	**Cholesterol:** 0 mg

INGREDIENTS:

1½ cups sliced fresh okra
½ cup chopped onion
½ cup chopped celery
½ teaspoon salt
¼ teaspoon pepper
⅛ teaspoon ground oregano

1 (16-ounce) can whole tomatoes, undrained and chopped
1 (7-ounce) can whole kernel corn, undrained

STEPS IN PREPARATION:

1. Combine all ingredients in a heavy nonstick skillet. Bring mixture to a boil.
2. Reduce heat; cover and simmer 15 to 20 minutes or until okra is tender.

Yield: 11 servings

OKRA FROM THE OVEN

Exchanges: 2 Vegetable

Serving Size: ½ cup	**Calories:** 44
Carbohydrate: 10 gm	**Fiber:** 4 gm
Protein: 2 gm	**Sodium:** 138 mg
Fat: trace	**Cholesterol:** 0 mg

INGREDIENTS:

3 cups sliced fresh okra
Vegetable cooking spray
1 cup chopped tomato
1 cup chopped onion

1 cup chopped green pepper
½ teaspoon salt
⅛ teaspoon pepper

STEPS IN PREPARATION:

1. Spread okra in a 13- x 9- x 2-inch baking dish coated with cooking spray.
2. Layer tomato, onion, and green pepper over okra. Sprinkle with salt and pepper.
3. Cover and bake at 400° for 1 hour or until okra is tender, stirring occasionally.

Yield: 8 servings

Fresh okra should have firm, bright green pods less than four inches long. To store, keep it in a plastic bag in the refrigerator for up to three days.

SKILLET OKRA

Exchanges: 1 Starch

Serving Size: ½ cup
Carbohyrate: 17 gm
Protein: 3 gm
Fat: 1 gm

Calories: 77
Fiber: 3 gm
Sodium: 283 mg
Cholesterol: 0 mg

INGREDIENTS:

1½ cups sliced fresh okra
½ cup chopped onion
½ cup chopped celery
¼ cup chopped green pepper
1 (16-ounce) can whole tomatoes, undrained and chopped

1 (16-ounce) can whole-kernel corn, undrained

STEPS IN PREPARATION:

1. Combine all ingredients in a large nonstick skillet, stirring well. Cover and bring to a boil.
2. Reduce heat, and simmer 15 to 20 minutes or until vegetables are tender.

Yield: 8 servings

PARMESAN PEAS

Exchanges: 1 Starch

Serving Size: ½ cup	**Calories:** 72
Carbohydrate: 12 gm	**Fiber:** 4 gm
Protein: 5 gm	**Sodium:** 96 mg
Fat: 1 gm	**Cholesterol:** trace

INGREDIENTS:

2 (10-ounce) packages frozen English peas
1 tablespoon grated Parmesan cheese
1 teaspoon lemon juice
1 teaspoon reduced-calorie margarine, melted
¼ teaspoon dried Italian seasoning
⅛ teaspoon grated lemon rind

STEPS IN PREPARATION:

1. Cook peas according to package directions, omitting salt and fat; drain.
2. Add cheese and remaining ingredients; toss to coat. Serve warm.

Yield: 6 servings

DILLY SQUASH

Exchanges: 1 Vegetable

Serving Size: ½ cup
Carbohydrate: 6 gm
Protein: 1 gm
Fat: trace

Calories: 27
Fiber: 2 gm
Sodium: 401 mg
Cholesterol: 0 mg

INGREDIENTS:

3 cups sliced yellow squash
1 teaspoon minced onion
1 tablespoon chopped fresh parsley

½ teaspoon salt
¼ teaspoon dried dillweed
1 tablespoon dry butter substitute

STEPS IN PREPARATION:

1. Arrange squash and onion in a vegetable steamer over boiling water. Cover and steam 5 minutes or until tender.
2. Remove from heat, and mash squash mixture.
3. Add parsley, salt, and dillweed; toss lightly.
4. Sprinkle with butter substitute, and serve warm.

Yield: 4 servings

Check the stems of yellow squash to determine its quality. If stems are hard, dry, shriveled, or darkened, the squash is not fresh.

BAKED SQUASH WITH ROSEMARY

Exchanges: 1 Vegetable, ½ Fat

Serving Size: 1 cup	**Calories:** 54
Carbohydrate: 8 gm	**Fiber:** 2 gm
Protein: 2 gm	**Sodium:** 13 mg
Fat: 2 gm	**Cholesterol:** trace

INGREDIENTS:

2 **pounds yellow squash**
1 **tablespoon low-sodium beef-flavored bouillon granules**
1 **cup hot water**

1 **teaspoon reduced-calorie margarine, melted**
½ **teaspoon dried rosemary, crushed**

STEPS IN PREPARATION:

1. Cut yellow squash in half lengthwise. Place squash halves, cut side down, in a large shallow baking dish.
2. Dissolve bouillon granules in hot water, and pour bouillon around squash in baking dish. Bake, uncovered, at 350° for 20 minutes.
3. Combine margarine and rosemary, stirring well.
4. Turn squash, and baste with margarine mixture. Bake, uncovered, 15 minutes or until squash is tender.

Yield: 6 servings

SQUASH CASSEROLE

Exchanges: 1 Vegetable, ½ Fat

Serving Size: ½ cup	**Calories:** 42
Carbohydrate: 4 gm	**Fiber:** 1 gm
Protein: 2 gm	**Sodium:** 360 mg
Fat: 2 gm	**Cholesterol:** 37 mg

INGREDIENTS:

1 pound yellow squash
½ cup chopped onion
¼ cup chopped green pepper
2 tablespoons reduced-calorie
   mayonnaise
1 teaspoon salt
2 (4-ounce) jars diced
   pimiento, drained

1 egg
Vegetable cooking spray
2 tablespoons cracker crumbs
¼ cup (1 ounce) shredded
   reduced-fat Cheddar cheese

STEPS IN PREPARATION:

1. Cook squash in boiling water to cover in a medium saucepan 15 minutes or until tender. Drain and mash.
2. Combine onion and next 5 ingredients in a medium bowl, stirring well. Stir in squash.
3. Spoon squash mixture into a 2-quart casserole coated with cooking spray. Sprinkle with cracker crumbs.
4. Bake at 325° for 25 minutes. Top with cheese, and bake an additional 5 minutes or until cheese melts.

Yield: 8 servings

BAKED ZUCCHINI SQUASH

Exchanges: 1 Vegetable

Serving Size: 2 squash halves
Carbohydrate: 11 gm
Protein: 2 gm
Fat: 1 gm

Calories: 53
Fiber: 2 gm
Sodium: 312 mg
Cholesterol: 1 mg

INGREDIENTS:

4 small zucchini, cut in half
   lengthwise
¼ cup plain low-fat yogurt
3 tablespoons minced onion
3 tablespoons chopped green
   pepper
Sugar substitute to equal 2
   teaspoons sugar*

¼ teaspoon salt
⅛ teaspoon ground allspice
⅛ teaspoon pepper
1 tablespoon dry butter
   substitute
4 saltine crackers, crushed

STEPS IN PREPARATION:

1. Cook zucchini in boiling water to cover in a medium saucepan 5 minutes or until crisp-tender. Drain well, and set aside.
2. Scoop out zucchini pulp, and place in a bowl; reserve zucchini shells.
3. Combine pulp, yogurt, and next 6 ingredients.
4. Spoon mixture into squash shells. Sprinkle with butter substitute and cracker crumbs. Bake at 350° for 30 minutes or until thoroughly heated.

Yield: 4 servings

*See the sugar substitution chart on page 354.

SAUTÉED ZUCCHINI

Exchanges: 1 Vegetable, ½ Fat

Serving Size: ½ cup
Carbohydrate: 8 gm
Protein: 3 gm
Fat: 2 gm

Calories: 53
Fiber: 2 gm
Sodium: 274 mg
Cholesterol: 3 mg

INGREDIENTS:

½ cup chopped onion
1 tablespoon reduced-calorie
  margarine, melted
3½ cups sliced zucchini
1 cup sliced mushrooms
½ teaspoon salt

½ teaspoon dried thyme
¼ teaspoon pepper
¼ cup (1 ounce) shredded
  low-fat process American
  cheese

STEPS IN PREPARATION:

1. Sauté onion in margarine in a nonstick skillet until tender.
2. Add zucchini and next 4 ingredients. Cook over low heat 5 to 7
   minutes or until zucchini is crisp-tender, stirring frequently.
3. Sprinkle with cheese, and serve immediately.

Yield: 6 servings

STUFFED BUTTERNUT SQUASH

Exchanges: ½ Starch

Serving Size: ½ cup	**Calories:** 55
Carbohydrate: 9 gm	**Fiber:** 2 gm
Protein: 2 gm	**Sodium:** 137 mg
Fat: 2 gm	**Cholesterol:** 1 mg

INGREDIENTS:

1 medium butternut squash
½ cup water
1 cup finely chopped apple
¼ cup chopped onion
2 teaspoons reduced-calorie margarine, melted
½ cup 1% low-fat cottage cheese

¼ teaspoon salt
⅛ teaspoon ground cinnamon
⅛ teaspoon ground ginger
⅛ teaspoon pepper
½ teaspoon apple pie spice

STEPS IN PREPARATION:

1. Cut squash in half lengthwise, and remove seeds. Place halves, cut side down, in an 11- x 7- x 2-inch baking dish. Pour water around squash, and bake at 350° for 45 minutes or until squash is tender.
2. Sauté apple and onion in margarine in a large nonstick skillet until onion is tender. Stir in cottage cheese and next 4 ingredients. Remove from heat, and set aside.
3. Carefully scoop out squash pulp, reserving shells. Chop pulp.
4. Add squash pulp to apple mixture in skillet, stirring well. Spoon mixture into squash shells, and sprinkle with apple pie spice. Bake at 375° for 15 minutes or until thoroughly heated.

Yield: 8 servings

STEWED TOMATOES

Exchanges: 1 Vegetable

Serving Size: ½ cup	**Calories:** 55
Carbohydrate: 9 gm	**Fiber:** 2 gm
Protein: 2 gm	**Sodium:** 350 mg
Fat: 1 gm	**Cholesterol:** 0 mg

INGREDIENTS:

1 tablespoon chopped green pepper
1 tablespoon chopped onion
1 tablespoon reduced-calorie margarine, melted
3 cups canned tomatoes, drained
2 slices white bread, cubed
¼ teaspoon salt
⅛ teaspoon black pepper

STEPS IN PREPARATION:

1. Sauté green pepper and onion in margarine in a medium nonstick skillet until tender.
2. Add tomato, bread, salt, and black pepper. Cook over medium heat until thoroughly heated, stirring occasionally.

Yield: 6 servings

SPINACH-STUFFED TOMATOES

Exchanges: 2 Vegetable

Serving Size: 1 stuffed tomato
Carbohydrate: 10 gm
Protein: 2 gm
Fat: 1 gm

Calories: 55
Fiber: 2 gm
Sodium: 191 mg
Cholesterol: trace

INGREDIENTS:

8 medium tomatoes
1 (10-ounce) package frozen chopped spinach, thawed
2 teaspoons reduced-calorie margarine
2 tablespoons all-purpose flour

½ teaspoon salt
½ teaspoon dry mustard
¼ teaspoon Worcestershire sauce
2 tablespoons soft breadcrumbs
Vegetable cooking spray

STEPS IN PREPARATION:

1. Cut tops from tomatoes; scoop out pulp, leaving shells intact. Chop pulp, and set aside. Invert tomato shells on paper towels; drain 10 minutes.
2. Cook spinach according to package directions, omitting salt and fat. Drain well.
3. Melt margarine in a medium saucepan over low heat; add flour, salt, mustard, and Worcestershire sauce, stirring until smooth. Cook, stirring constantly, 1 minute. Stir in tomato pulp and spinach. Remove from heat.
4. Spoon spinach mixture into tomato shells. Top with breadcrumbs, and place in a shallow baking dish coated with cooking spray. Bake at 400° for 15 minutes or until mixture is thoroughly heated and breadcrumbs are lightly browned.

Yield: 8 servings

BAKED TOMATOES

Exchanges: 1 Vegetable

Serving Size: 2 tomato halves
Carbohydrate: 11 gm
Protein: 2 gm
Fat: 1 gm

Calories: 56
Fiber: 1 gm
Sodium: 193 mg
Cholesterol: 0 mg

INGREDIENTS:

4 medium tomatoes, cut in
   half
Vegetable cooking spray
¼ teaspoon salt
⅛ teaspoon pepper
¼ cup soft breadcrumbs,
   toasted

3 tablespoons minced fresh
   parsley
¼ teaspoon dried thyme
¼ teaspoon dried oregano
⅛ teaspoon garlic powder
Fresh parsley sprigs (optional)

STEPS IN PREPARATION:

1. Place tomato halves, cut side up, in an 11- x 7- x 2-inch baking
   dish coated with cooking spray. Sprinkle with salt and pepper.
2. Combine breadcrumbs and next 4 ingredients; stir well.
3. Spoon mixture evenly over tomato halves. Bake at 350° for 12 to
   15 minutes or until thoroughly heated. Garnish with parsley
   sprigs, if desired.

Yield: 4 servings

SCALLOPED TOMATOES

Exchanges: 1 Vegetable

Serving Size: ½ cup	**Calories:** 70
Carbohydrate: 14 gm	**Fiber:** 1 gm
Protein: 2 gm	**Sodium:** 580 mg
Fat: 1 gm	**Cholesterol:** 1 mg

INGREDIENTS:

1 (20-ounce) can tomatoes
1 beef bouillon cube
1 cup cubed white bread
2 tablespoons chopped onion
2 tablespoons chopped celery

½ teaspoon salt
2 tablespoons dry butter
   substitute
Vegetable cooking spray

STEPS IN PREPARATION:

1. Drain tomatoes, reserving liquid. Pour tomato liquid into a medium saucepan; bring to a boil. Add bouillon cube, stirring to dissolve.
2. Add tomato, bread, and next 3 ingredients. Sprinkle with butter substitute.
3. Transfer to a 1-quart casserole coated with cooking spray. Bake at 400° for 25 minutes or until thoroughly heated.

Yield: 8 servings

TURNIP GREENS

Exchanges: 2 Vegetable

Serving Size: ½ cup	**Calories:** 51
Carbohydrate: 10 gm	**Fiber:** 5 gm
Protein: 2 gm	**Sodium:** 273 mg
Fat: 1 gm	**Cholesterol:** 0 mg

INGREDIENTS:

2 **pounds fresh turnip greens**
3 **cups water**
½ **teaspoon salt**
½ **cup chopped onion**
2 **teaspoons reduced-calorie margarine, melted**
⅛ **teaspoon ground allspice**
1 **tablespoon all-purpose flour**
Sugar substitute to equal 1 teaspoon sugar*
2 **tablespoons vinegar**

STEPS IN PREPARATION:

1. Combine first 3 ingredients in large Dutch oven; bring to a boil. Reduce heat; simmer 1 hour or until tender.
2. Drain greens, reserving 1 cup liquid; set aside.
3. Sauté onion in margarine in a nonstick skillet. Add sautéed onion and allspice to drained greens.
4. Stir flour and sugar substitute into vinegar, stirring to dissolve; add to reserved 1 cup liquid. Add flour mixture to greens.
5. Cook over medium heat until thickened, stirring occasionally.

Yield: 6 servings

*See the sugar substitution chart on page 354.

MIXED VEGETABLE CASSEROLE

Exchanges: 2 Vegetable, ½ Fat

Serving Size: ½ cup	**Calories:** 66
Carbohydrate: 9 gm	**Fiber:** 2 gm
Protein: 3 gm	**Sodium:** 140 mg
Fat: 2 gm	**Cholesterol:** 4 mg

INGREDIENTS:

2 (10-ounce) packages frozen mixed vegetables

½ cup (2 ounces) shredded low-fat process American cheese

2 tablespoons chopped onion

2 tablespoons reduced-calorie mayonnaise

1 (8-ounce) can sliced water chestnuts, drained

Vegetable cooking spray

STEPS IN PREPARATION:

1. Cook mixed vegetables according to package directions, omitting salt and fat. Drain.
2. Combine mixed vegetables, cheese, and next 3 ingredients, stirring gently.
3. Spoon mixture into a 1½-quart casserole coated with cooking spray. Bake at 350° for 20 minutes or until thoroughly heated.

Yield: 8 servings

STIR-FRIED VEGETABLES

Exchanges: 1 Vegetable

Serving Size: 1 cup	**Calories:** 41
Carbohydrate: 8 gm	**Fiber:** 1 gm
Protein: 2 gm	**Sodium:** 80 mg
Fat: trace	**Cholesterol:** trace

INGREDIENTS:

Vegetable cooking spray
1 tablespoon reduced-sodium soy sauce
1 clove garlic, crushed
3 cups shredded cabbage
2 cups broccoli flowerets
1 cup sliced carrot
1 cup sliced green onions
2 cups sliced fresh mushrooms
1 (6-ounce) package frozen snow pea pods, thawed
1 cup water
1 tablespoon cornstarch
2 teaspoons chicken-flavored bouillon granules

STEPS IN PREPARATION:

1. Coat a wok or large nonstick skillet with cooking spray. Heat at medium-high (375°) until hot. Add soy sauce and garlic; stir-fry 3 minutes.
2. Add cabbage, broccoli, carrot, and green onions. Stir-fry 3 to 4 minutes or until vegetables are crisp-tender.
3. Add mushrooms and snow peas; stir-fry 2 minutes.
4. Combine water, cornstarch, and bouillon granules, stirring to dissolve. Pour over vegetable mixture, and stir-fry until thickened and bubbly.

Yield: 8 servings

MARINATED GARDEN VEGETABLES

Exchanges: 1 Vegetable, ½ Fat

Serving Size: ½ cup
Carbohydrate: 7 gm
Protein: 1 gm
Fat: 2 gm

Calories: 52
Fiber: 2 gm
Sodium: 310 mg
Cholesterol: 1 mg

INGREDIENTS:

2 cups broccoli flowerets
2 cups cauliflower flowerets
2 cups sliced carrot
½ cup chopped green pepper
½ cup sliced celery
1 medium zucchini, sliced

1 medium cucumber, sliced
Garden Vegetable Marinade
  (page 295)
4 small tomatoes, cut into
  quarters
1 cup sliced fresh mushrooms

STEPS IN PREPARATION:

1. Combine first 7 ingredients in a large bowl.
2. Pour Garden Vegetable Marinade over vegetables. Toss gently to coat.
3. Cover and marinate in refrigerator at least 12 hours, stirring occasionally. (Mixture can be stored in refrigerator up to 1 week.)
4. Add tomato and mushrooms just before serving.

Yield: 20 servings

Salads and
Salad
Dressings

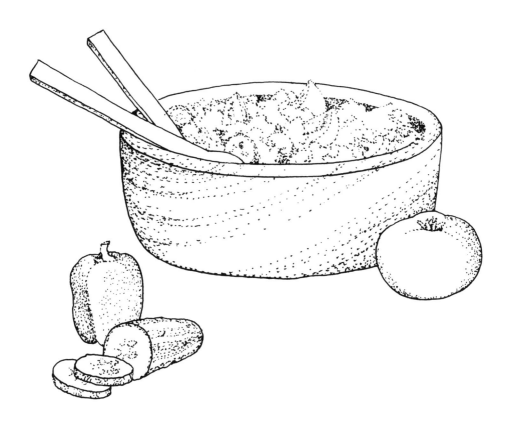

WALDORF SALAD

Exchanges: 1 Fruit, 1 Fat

Serving Size: ½ cup
Carbohydrate: 10 gm
Protein: trace
Fat: 4 gm

Calories: 151
Fiber: 2 gm
Sodium: 70 mg
Cholesterol: 0 mg

INGREDIENTS:

3 medium-size Red Delicious
  apples, cored and diced
½ cup sliced celery
¼ cup raisins

½ cup reduced-calorie
  mayonnaise
1 tablespoon lemon juice

STEPS IN PREPARATION:

1. Combine apple, celery, and raisins in a medium bowl.
2. Combine mayonnaise and lemon juice, stirring well. Add mayonaise mixture to fruit mixture, and toss lightly to coat.
3. Cover and chill.

Yield: 5 servings

Planning meals? Remember fruit salads are as satisfying as vegetable salads and can be used for any brunch, lunch, or dinner menu.

MIXED FRUIT SALAD

Exchanges: 1 Fruit

Serving Size: ⅓ cup
Carbohydrate: 15 gm
Protein: trace
Fat: trace

Calories: 57
Fiber: 1 gm
Sodium: 92 mg
Cholesterol: 0 mg

INGREDIENTS:

1 cup chopped apple
1 cup sliced banana
½ cup raisins
½ cup chopped celery
⅓ cup reduced-calorie
   mayonnaise

1 tablespoon lemon juice
1 (8-ounce) can pineapple
   chunks in juice, drained
Lettuce leaves (optional)

STEPS IN PREPARATION:

1. Combine first 7 ingredients in a medium bowl; toss gently to coat.
2. Cover and chill 1 hour.
3. Serve on lettuce leaves, if desired.

Yield: 16 servings

FRESH FRUIT SALAD

Exchanges: 1 Fruit

Serving Size: ½ cup
Carbohydrate: 9 gm
Protein: 1 gm
Fat: 1 gm

Calories: 47
Fiber: 1 gm
Sodium: 82 mg
Cholesterol: 0 mg

INGREDIENTS:

½ cup sliced fresh
  strawberries
½ cup seedless green grapes,
  cut in half
½ small cantaloupe, diced
¼ cup plain nonfat yogurt
2 tablespoons nonfat
  mayonnaise

1 tablespoon granulated
  brown sugar substitute
1 tablespoon chopped
  walnuts
Lettuce leaves (optional)

STEPS IN PREPARATION:

1. Combine strawberries, grapes, and cantaloupe.
2. Combine yogurt, mayonnaise, brown sugar substitute, and nuts,
   stirring well. Stir yogurt mixture into fruit mixture.
3. Serve on lettuce leaves, if desired.

Yield: 6 servings

CONGEALED PEACH SALAD

Exchanges: 1 Fruit

Serving Size: 1 cup
Carbohydrate: 5 gm
Protein: 7 gm
Fat: 2 gm

Calories: 74
Fiber: 1 gm
Sodium: 235 mg
Cholesterol: 0 mg

INGREDIENTS:

1 (16-ounce) can peach slices
  in juice, drained
Vegetable cooking spray
2 (3-ounce) packages
  sugar-free orange or lemon
  gelatin

1½ cups boiling water
1 (12-ounce) can sugar-free
  ginger ale
¼ cup chopped walnuts

STEPS IN PREPARATION:

1. Set aside ½ cup peach slices. Arrange remaining peaches in bottom of a 1½-quart mold coated with cooking spray, overlapping slices.
2. Dissolve gelatin in boiling water; add ginger ale, and chill until slightly thickened. Beat gelatin mixture until fluffy.
3. Chop reserved ½ cup peach slices, and fold into gelatin. Fold in walnuts. Spoon gelatin mixture over peaches in mold.
4. Cover and chill at least 8 hours.
5. To serve, unmold onto a serving platter.

Yield: 8 servings

PINEAPPLE-ORANGE SALAD

Exchanges: 1 Fruit

Serving Size: ¼ cup
Carbohydrate: 15 gm
Protein: 2 gm
Fat: trace

Calories: 64
Fiber: 1 gm
Sodium: 49 mg
Cholesterol: 0 mg

INGREDIENTS:

- 2 envelopes unflavored gelatin
- 2 cups unsweetened orange juice, divided
- 2 cups canned crushed pineapple in juice, drained

Sugar substitute to equal ¼ cup sugar*
- 2 tablespoons lemon juice
- ½ teaspoon almond extract
- ¼ teaspoon salt
- Vegetable cooking spray

STEPS IN PREPARATION:

1. Sprinkle gelatin over ½ cup orange juice to soften.
2. Heat remaining 1½ cups orange juice, and pour over softened gelatin mixture; stir until gelatin is dissolved.
3. Add pineapple and next 4 ingredients; stir well. Pour into a 3-cup mold coated with cooking spray; chill until set.
4. To serve, unmold onto a serving platter.

Yield: 12 servings

*See the sugar substitution chart on page 354.

PINEAPPLE-LIME SALAD

Exchanges: ½ Skim Milk

Serving Size: ½ cup
Carbohydrate: 5 gm
Protein: 5 gm
Fat: 1 gm

Calories: 50
Fiber: trace
Sodium: 112 mg
Cholesterol: 2 mg

INGREDIENTS:

1 (0.6-ounce) package sugar-free lime-flavored gelatin
2 cups boiling water
2 cups cold water
2 tablespoons reduced-calorie mayonnaise

1 cup 1% low-fat cottage cheese
1 (8¼-ounce) can crushed pineapple in juice, drained
Vegetable cooking spray
Lettuce leaves (optional)

STEPS IN PREPARATION:

1. Dissolve gelatin in boiling water in a medium bowl, stirring well. Stir in cold water. Chill until mixture is the consistency of unbeaten egg white.
2. Fold mayonnaise into gelatin mixture. Add cottage cheese and pineapple, stirring well.
3. Pour gelatin mixture into a 6-cup mold coated with cooking spray; chill gelatin mixture until set.
4. To serve, unmold onto lettuce leaves, if desired.

Yield: 10 servings

STRAWBERRY SALAD

Exchanges: 1 Fruit

Serving Size: ½ cup
Carbohydrate: 9 gm
Protein: 5 gm
Fat: trace

Calories: 60
Fiber: 1 gm
Sodium: 93 mg
Cholesterol: 1 mg

INGREDIENTS:

1 (3-ounce) package sugar-free strawberry gelatin
¾ cup chopped fresh strawberries
1 cup plain nonfat yogurt

Sugar substitute to equal 2 teaspoons sugar*
1 teaspoon vanilla extract
Vegetable cooking spray

STEPS IN PREPARATION:

1. Prepare gelatin according to package directions. Chill until slightly thickened.
2. Mash strawberries; add to gelatin mixture. Add yogurt, sugar substitute, and vanilla; stir until well blended.
3. Pour into 4 (½-cup) molds coated with cooking spray; chill until set.
4. To serve, unmold onto salad plates.

Yield: 4 servings

*See the sugar substitution chart on page 354.

CONGEALED VEGETABLE SALAD

Exchanges: Free

Serving Size: ½ cup	**Calories:** 14
Carbohydrate: 2 gm	**Fiber:** trace
Protein: 2 gm	**Sodium:** 18 mg
Fat: trace	**Cholesterol:** 0 mg

INGREDIENTS:

1 (0.6-ounce) package sugar-free lime-flavored gelatin
2 cups boiling water
1¾ cups cold water
¼ cup vinegar
1 cup chopped celery
1 cup shredded carrot
2 tablespoons chopped sweet red pepper
2 tablespoons chopped green onions
Vegetable cooking spray
Lettuce leaves (optional)

STEPS IN PREPARATION:

1. Dissolve gelatin in boiling water in a medium bowl, stirring well. Stir in cold water and vinegar. Chill until mixture is the consistency of unbeaten egg white.
2. Fold in vegetables, and pour gelatin mixture into 10 (½-cup) molds coated with cooking spray. Chill until set.
3. To serve, unmold onto lettuce leaves, if desired.

Yield: 10 servings

PICKLED BEET SALAD

Exchanges: 1 Vegetable

Serving Size: ½ cup
Carbohydrate: 9 gm
Protein: 1 gm
Fat: trace

Calories: 35
Fiber: 2 gm
Sodium: 256 mg
Cholesterol: 0 mg

INGREDIENTS:

3 cups canned beets in juice
¼ cup vinegar
Sugar substitute to equal 2
   tablespoons sugar*

½ teaspoon salt
¼ teaspoon ground cinnamon
⅛ teaspoon ground cloves
Dash of pepper

STEPS IN PREPARATION:

1. Drain beets, and place in a medium bowl; reserve juice in a saucepan.
2. Add vinegar and remaining ingredients to beet juice. Bring juice mixture to a boil; immediately remove from heat.
3. Pour juice mixture over beets.
4. Cover and chill; drain beets before serving.

Yield: 6 servings

*See the sugar substitution chart on page 354.

GREEN BEAN SALAD

Exchanges: 1 Vegetable, 1 Fat

Serving Size: ½ cup
Carbohydrate: 9 gm
Protein: 1 gm
Fat: 6 gm

Calories: 89
Fiber: 5 gm
Sodium: 880 mg
Cholesterol: 4 mg

INGREDIENTS:

- 2 (10-ounce) cans cut green beans, undrained
- 1 cup commercial no-oil Italian dressing
- ½ cup chopped dill pickles
- ½ teaspoon dried basil
- ½ teaspoon dried oregano
- 1 small red onion, sliced
- 1 clove garlic, minced

STEPS IN PREPARATION:

1. Place beans in a medium saucepan; cook over medium heat 5 minutes or until thoroughly heated. Drain.
2. Combine beans, Italian dressing, and remaining ingredients in a medium bowl; toss lightly to coat.
3. Cover and chill at least 8 hours.
4. Serve with a slotted spoon.

Yield: 4 servings

If you want to reduce sodium, use canned no-salt-added cut green beans in this recipe and others.

CARROT-RAISIN SALAD

Exchanges: 1 Fruit, 1 Vegetable

Serving Size: ¼ cup	**Calories:** 86
Carbohydrate: 20 gm	**Fiber:** 2 gm
Protein: 3 gm	**Sodium:** 39 mg
Fat: trace	**Cholesterol:** 1 mg

INGREDIENTS:

2 cups shredded carrot
1 cup canned crushed
   pineapple in juice, drained
½ cup raisins

1 (8-ounce) carton plain
   nonfat yogurt
Lettuce leaves (optional)

STEPS IN PREPARATION:

1. Combine carrot, pineapple, and raisins; stir well.
2. Cover and chill at least 2 hours.
3. Stir in yogurt, and serve on lettuce leaves, if desired.

Yield: 12 servings

CHILLED CAULIFLOWER SALAD

Exchanges: 1 Vegetable

Serving Size: ½ cup
Carbohydrate: 4 gm
Protein: 1 gm
Fat: 1 gm

Calories: 29
Fiber: 1 gm
Sodium: 170 mg
Cholesterol: 1 mg

INGREDIENTS:

1 medium cauliflower, broken into flowerets
½ cup sliced celery
½ cup commercial no-oil Italian dressing
¼ teaspoon salt
¼ teaspoon black pepper
¼ teaspoon ground red pepper
2 small cloves garlic, minced

STEPS IN PREPARATION:

1. Place cauliflower and water to cover in a medium saucepan; cover and bring to a boil. Cook 4 to 5 minutes or until crisp-tender. Drain.
2. Combine cooked cauliflower and celery in a medium bowl.
3. Combine Italian dressing and remaining ingredients, stirring well. Pour dressing mixture over cauliflower mixture, tossing gently to coat.
4. Cover and chill at least 2 hours.

Yield: 10 servings

MARINATED CUCUMBER SALAD

Exchanges: 1 Vegetable

Serving Size: ½ cup	**Calories:** 35
Carbohydrate: 3 gm	**Fiber:** 1 gm
Protein: trace	**Sodium:** 192 mg
Fat: 2 gm	**Cholesterol:** 1 mg

INGREDIENTS:

½ cup commercial no-oil
  Italian dressing
⅛ teaspoon pepper
1 medium cucumber, peeled
  and thinly sliced

½ small onion, thinly sliced
¼ cup thinly sliced radishes
2 tablespoons chopped fresh
  parsley

STEPS IN PREPARATION:

1. Combine Italian dressing and pepper in a medium bowl, stirring well. Add cucumber, onion, radishes, and parsley. Toss gently to coat.
2. Cover and marinate in refrigerator at least 4 hours.
3. Serve with a slotted spoon.

Yield: 5 servings

Add marinated vegetable salads to your next dinner party menu. They can be prepared in advance and chilled until serving time—an important time-saver for busy cooks.

COLESLAW

Exchanges: 1 Vegetable

Serving Size: ½ cup	**Calories:** 23
Carbohydrate: 5 gm	**Fiber:** 1 gm
Protein: 1 gm	**Sodium:** 316 mg
Fat: trace	**Cholesterol:** 0 mg

INGREDIENTS:

4 cups shredded cabbage
½ cup shredded carrot
⅓ cup nonfat mayonnaise
2 tablespoons prepared
   mustard

2 tablespoons vinegar
½ teaspoon salt

STEPS IN PREPARATION:

1. Combine all ingredients in a medium bowl. Toss gently to coat.
2. Cover and chill.

Yield: 8 servings

Select cabbage with fresh, crisp leaves that are firmly packed and a head that is heavy for its size. Cabbage will keep in the refrigerator, tightly wrapped in heavy-duty plastic wrap, for about two weeks.

CALIFORNIA COLESLAW

Exchanges: 1 Vegetable

Serving Size: ½ cup	**Calories:** 22
Carbohydrate: 4 gm	**Fiber:** 1 gm
Protein: trace	**Sodium:** 103 mg
Fat: 1 gm	**Cholesterol:** trace

INGREDIENTS:

1 cup shredded cabbage
1 cup shredded red cabbage
½ cup shredded carrot
½ cup chopped green pepper
½ cup chopped sweet red pepper
¼ cup chopped onion
1½ tablespoons minced fresh parsley

¼ cup vinegar
¼ cup commercial no-oil Italian dressing
Liquid sugar substitute to equal ¼ cup sugar*
⅛ teaspoon salt
⅛ teaspoon pepper

STEPS IN PREPARATION:

1. Combine first 7 ingredients in a large bowl, stirring well. Set aside.
2. Combine vinegar and remaining ingredients in a jar; cover tightly, and shake vigorously.
3. Pour dressing mixture over vegetables, tossing gently to coat.
4. Cover and chill.
5. To serve, stir coleslaw lightly, and serve with a slotted spoon.

Yield: 8 servings

*See the sugar substitution chart on page 354.

MARINATED COLESLAW

Exchanges: 1 Vegetable, ½ Fat

Serving Size: ½ cup	**Calories:** 59
Carbohydrate: 7 gm	**Fiber:** 2 gm
Protein: 1 gm	**Sodium:** 241 mg
Fat: 3 gm	**Cholesterol:** 2 mg

INGREDIENTS:

3 cups shredded cabbage
Sugar substitute to equal ¾
   cup sugar*
1 large green pepper, diced
1 large onion, diced

1½ cups commercial no-oil
   Italian dressing
1 tablespoon celery seeds
1 tablespoon dry mustard

STEPS IN PREPARATION:

1. Combine first 4 ingredients in a large bowl; stir well.
2. Combine Italian dressing, celery seeds, and dry mustard in a small saucepan. Bring to a boil, and remove from heat.
3. Pour dressing mixture over vegetable mixture, tossing gently to coat.
4. Cover and chill at least 1 hour.
5. To serve, stir coleslaw lightly, and serve with a slotted spoon.

Yield: 12 servings

*See the sugar substitution chart on page 354.

MARINATED VEGETABLE SALAD

Exchanges: 1 Vegetable

Serving Size: ½ cup
Carbohydrate: 11 gm
Protein: 1 gm
Fat: 1 gm

Calories: 56
Fiber: 2 gm
Sodium: 119 mg
Cholesterol: 1 mg

INGREDIENTS:

3 cups diagonally sliced
  carrot
1 cup chopped celery
½ cup chopped green pepper
1 teaspoon celery seeds
1 medium onion, thinly sliced

Sugar substitute to equal 1
  cup sugar*
½ cup commercial no-oil
  Italian salad dressing
¼ cup vinegar
¼ cup water

STEPS IN PREPARATION:

1. Place carrot in a small saucepan; cover with water, and boil 10 minutes or until crisp-tender. Drain well.
2. Place carrot, celery, and next 3 ingredients in a large shallow dish; toss lightly, and set aside.
3. Combine sugar substitute and remaining ingredients in a small saucepan, stirring well; bring to a boil, stirring frequently. Pour mixture over vegetables.
4. Cover and chill at least 8 hours.

Yield: 10 servings

*See the sugar substitution chart on page 354.

MACARONI SALAD

Exchanges: 1½ Starch, ½ Fat

Serving Size: ½ cup
Carbohydrate: 21 gm
Protein: 5 gm
Fat: 3 gm

Calories: 133
Fiber: 1 gm
Sodium: 366 mg
Cholesterol: 48 mg

INGREDIENTS:

1½ cups elbow macaroni, uncooked
¼ cup chopped green onions
2 hard-cooked eggs, chopped
2 dill pickles, chopped
½ cup commercial no-oil Italian dressing

2 tablespoons dill pickle juice
1 tablespoon prepared mustard
1 teaspoon dried dillweed

STEPS IN PREPARATION:

1. Cook macaroni according to package directions, omitting salt and fat. Drain well. Combine macaroni, onions, eggs, and chopped pickle in a large bowl.
2. Combine Italian dressing and remaining ingredients, stirring to blend. Pour over macaroni mixture; stir well to coat.
3. Cover and chill at least 1 hour.

Yield: 8 servings

POTATO SALAD

Exchanges: 1 Starch, ½ Medium-Fat Meat

Serving Size: ½ cup	**Calories:** 99
Carbohydrate: 15 gm	**Fiber:** 1 gm
Protein: 4 gm	**Sodium:** 243 mg
Fat: 3 gm	**Cholesterol:** 94 mg

INGREDIENTS:

2 medium baking potatoes
2 tablespoons diced celery
2 tablespoons prepared mustard
2 tablespoons reduced-calorie mayonnaise
2 teaspoons chopped onion
2 teaspoons chopped green pepper
2 teaspoons diced pimiento
2 teaspoons chopped dill pickle
2 hard-cooked eggs, chopped

STEPS IN PREPARATION:

1. Cook potatoes in boiling water to cover 30 minutes or until tender. Drain and cool slightly. Peel and dice potatoes.
2. Combine potato, celery, and remaining ingredients in a medium bowl, tossing to coat.
3. Cover and chill at least 1 hour.

Yield: 4 servings

TARRAGON POTATO SALAD

Exchanges: 1 Starch

Serving Size: ½ cup
Carbohydrate: 16 gm
Protein: 2 gm
Fat: 1 gm

Calories: 84
Fiber: 2 gm
Sodium: 124 mg
Cholesterol: 1 mg

INGREDIENTS:

1⅓ pounds round red
   potatoes, unpeeled
¾ teaspoon dried tarragon
½ teaspoon dried parsley
   flakes
½ teaspoon dry mustard

1 small clove garlic
½ cup commercial no-oil
   Italian dressing
¾ teaspoon lemon juice
2 tablespoons minced green
   onions

STEPS IN PREPARATION:

1. Cook potatoes in boiling water to cover 15 minutes or until tender. Drain well, and cool. Cut into ¼-inch slices, and set aside.
2. Combine tarragon, parsley, mustard, and garlic in container of an electric blender. Cover and process 30 seconds or until pureed. Add Italian dressing, and process until blended. With blender running, slowly add lemon juice, and continue to process dressing mixture until smooth.
3. Add dressing mixture to cooked potato slices; add minced green onions, and toss well to coat.
4. Cover and chill.

Yield: 8 servings

TOMATO ASPIC

Exchanges: 1 Vegetable

Serving Size: ½ cup
Carbohydrate: 7 gm
Protein: 3 gm
Fat: trace

Calories: 35
Fiber: 1 gm
Sodium: 776 mg
Cholesterol: 0 mg

INGREDIENTS:

3 cups tomato juice
1 teaspoon salt
⅛ teaspoon pepper
2 lemon slices
1 stalk celery, sliced
1 small onion, sliced
1 bay leaf

⅔ cup chilled tomato juice
¼ cup vinegar
2 envelopes unflavored gelatin
¼ cup finely chopped celery
Vegetable cooking spray

Lettuce leaves (optional)

STEPS IN PREPARATION:

1. Combine first 7 ingredients in a medium saucepan. Simmer, uncovered, for 10 minutes. Strain mixture; remove and discard lemon slices, celery, onion, and bay leaf. Set aside, and keep warm.
2. Combine ⅔ cup tomato juice and vinegar; sprinkle gelatin over mixture to soften. Add warm juice mixture, stirring until gelatin dissolves.
3. Cover and chill until mixture begins to thicken.
4. Stir in chopped celery. Pour mixture into 7 (½-cup) molds coated with cooking spray; chill until set.
5. To serve, unmold on lettuce leaves, if desired.

Yield: 7 servings

SPINACH-MANDARIN SALAD

Exchanges: 1 Lean Meat, 1 Vegetable

Serving Size: 1 cup	**Calories:** 87
Carbohydrate: 6 gm	**Fiber:** 2 gm
Protein: 9 gm	**Sodium:** 317 mg
Fat: 3 gm	**Cholesterol:** 17 mg

INGREDIENTS:

4 cups fresh spinach
2 cups cherry tomatoes
1½ cups chopped cooked chicken breast (skinned before cooking and cooked without salt), chilled
1 cup thinly sliced radishes
½ pound fresh mushrooms, sliced
½ cup commercial croutons
Mandarin Dressing (page 282)
2 tablespoons sesame seeds, toasted

STEPS IN PREPARATION:

1. Wash spinach leaves thoroughly in cold water; drain. Remove and discard stems.
2. Place spinach in a large bowl. Add tomatoes and next 4 ingredients.
3. Add Mandarin Dressing, and toss gently. Top with sesame seeds.

Yield: 10 servings

CHEF'S SALAD

Exchanges: 1 Lean Meat, 1 Vegetable

Serving Size: 1½ cups	**Calories:** 81
Carbohydrate: 5 gm	**Fiber:** 1 gm
Protein: 8 gm	**Sodium:** 262 mg
Fat: 4 gm	**Cholesterol:** 38 mg

INGREDIENTS:

8 cups torn iceberg lettuce
1 cup thinly sliced radishes
2 green onions, sliced
⅓ cup Thousand Island Dressing (page 283)
2 ounces chopped lean cooked ham
2 ounces chopped cooked turkey breast

2 (1-ounce) slices low-fat process American cheese, diced
1 (1-ounce) slice low-fat Swiss cheese, diced
2 small tomatoes, chopped
1 hard-cooked egg, chopped

STEPS IN PREPARATION:

1. Combine first 3 ingredients in a large bowl. Cover and chill.
2. Pour Thousand Island Dressing over vegetable mixture; toss gently to coat. Top with ham and remaining ingredients.

Yield: 8 servings

TURKEY SALAD

Exchanges: 1 Lean Meat, 1 Vegetable

Serving Size: 1 cup
Carbohydrate: 5 gm
Protein: 10 gm
Fat: 4 gm

Calories: 97
Fiber: 2 gm
Sodium: 487 mg
Cholesterol: 77 mg

INGREDIENTS:

2 cups chopped fresh spinach
5 ounces cooked turkey, cut into ½-inch strips
1 (10½-ounce) can asparagus spears, drained and chopped
2 medium tomatoes, sliced
2 hard-cooked eggs, chopped
1 green onion, chopped
¼ cup plus 2 tablespoons commercial no-oil Italian dressing
¼ cup prepared mustard

STEPS IN PREPARATION:

1. Combine first 6 ingredients in a large bowl. Cover and chill.
2. Combine Italian dressing and mustard, stirring until blended. Pour over salad, and toss gently to coat.
3. Cover and chill.

Yield: 6 servings

You don't have to cook an entire bird to enjoy the flavor of turkey. Check your local supermarket for small cuts such as turkey breast slices, tenderloins, or boneless turkey breast roasts.

CUCUMBER DRESSING

Exchanges: Free

Serving Size: 2 tablespoons
Carbohydrate: 2 gm
Protein: 1 gm
Fat: trace

Calories: 18
Fiber: trace
Sodium: 156 mg
Cholesterol: trace

INGREDIENTS:

1 small cucumber, peeled
½ teaspoon salt
½ cup plain low-fat yogurt
1 tablespoon reduced-calorie mayonnaise

¼ teaspoon lemon juice
1 tablespoon chopped fresh parsley
1 green onion, chopped
¼ teaspoon dried dillweed

STEPS IN PREPARATION:

1. Shred cucumber; spread on a paper towel. Sprinkle with salt. Let stand at room temperature 30 minutes. Squeeze excess moisture from cucumber.
2. Combine yogurt, mayonnaise, and lemon juice in a small bowl, stirring to blend. Stir in drained cucumber, parsley, green onion, and dillweed.
3. Cover and chill. Stir well before using.
4. Serve with salad greens.

Yield: 1 cup

Note: See the Vegetable List on page 22 for exchange values of salad greens.

FRENCH DRESSING

Exchanges: 1 Fat

Serving Size: 2 tablespoons
Carbohydrate: 3 gm
Protein: trace
Fat: 5 gm

Calories: 60
Fiber: trace
Sodium: 201 mg
Cholesterol: 0 mg

INGREDIENTS:

3 tablespoons vegetable oil
¾ teaspoon salt
½ teaspoon dry mustard
¼ teaspoon hot sauce

⅛ teaspoon paprika
1 cup unsweetened grapefruit
  juice, divided
2 teaspoons cornstarch

STEPS IN PREPARATION:

1. Combine first 5 ingredients in a small bowl, stirring well to blend. Set aside.
2. Combine ½ cup grapefruit juice and cornstarch in a small saucepan, stirring until blended. Cook over medium heat, stirring constantly, until mixture is thickened and bubbly. Remove from heat.
3. Add cornstarch mixture to oil mixture in bowl, and beat at medium speed of an electric mixer until smooth. Add remaining ½ cup grapefruit juice, and beat until dressing mixture is well blended.
4. Cover and chill.
5. Serve with salad greens.

Yield: 1 cup

Note: See the Vegetable List on page 22 for exchange values of salad greens.

HERB DRESSING
Exchanges: Free

Serving Size: 2 tablespoons
Carbohydrate: 2 gm
Protein: trace
Fat: 0 gm

Calories: 12
Fiber: 0 gm
Sodium: 0 mg
Cholesterol: 0 mg

INGREDIENTS:

½ cup white wine vinegar
¼ cup salad vinegar
1 teaspoon onion powder

1 teaspoon dried salad herbs
1 teaspoon lemon juice
½ teaspoon garlic powder

STEPS IN PREPARATION:

1. Combine all ingredients in a jar; cover tightly, and shake vigorously. Chill.
2. Shake well before using.
3. Serve with salad greens.

Yield: ¾ cup

Note: See the Vegetable List on page 22 for exchange values of salad greens.

ITALIAN DRESSING

Exchanges: 1 Fat

Serving Size: 2 tablespoons
Carbohydrate: 1 gm
Protein: trace
Fat: 5 gm

Calories: 49
Fiber: trace
Sodium: 111 mg
Cholesterol: 1 mg

INGREDIENTS:

¼ cup plus 2 tablespoons water
¼ cup vinegar
2 tablespoons chopped fresh parsley
2 tablespoons vegetable oil
1 tablespoon plus 1 teaspoon grated Parmesan cheese

2 teaspoons dry pectin
¼ teaspoon salt
¼ teaspoon pepper
¼ teaspoon dried Italian seasoning
1 large clove garlic, peeled

STEPS IN PREPARATION:

1. Combine first 9 ingredients in a jar; cover tightly, and shake vigorously.
2. Press a wooden pick through garlic clove; add garlic clove to dressing mixture. Cover and chill.
3. To serve, remove and discard garlic. Cover and shake well before using.
4. Serve with salad greens.

Yield: ¾ cup

Note: See the Vegetable List on page 22 for exchange values of salad greens.

MANDARIN DRESSING

Exchanges: ½ Fat

Serving Size: 2 tablespoons
Carbohydrate: 4 gm
Protein: 1 gm
Fat: 3 gm

Calories: 42
Fiber: 1 gm
Sodium: 558 mg
Cholesterol: 1 mg

INGREDIENTS:

¼ cup commercial no-oil
  Italian dressing
Sugar substitute to equal 2
  tablespoons sugar*
2 tablespoons reduced-sodium
  soy sauce

1 teaspoon vinegar
1 teaspoon sesame seeds
⅛ teaspoon pepper

STEPS IN PREPARATION:

1. Combine all ingredients in a jar; cover tightly, and shake vigorously.
2. Chill at least 2 hours to blend flavors.
3. Serve over vegetable salads.

Yield: ¼ cup plus 2 tablespoons

Note: See the Vegetable List on page 22 for exchange values of vegetables.

*See the sugar substitution chart on page 354.

THOUSAND ISLAND DRESSING

Exchanges: ½ Fat

Serving Size: 2 tablespoons
Carbohydrate: 2 gm
Protein: 1 gm
Fat: 1 gm

Calories: 21
Fiber: trace
Sodium: 109 mg
Cholesterol: trace

INGREDIENTS:

¼ **cup plain low-fat yogurt**
¼ **cup nonfat buttermilk**
1 **tablespoon reduced-calorie mayonnaise**
1 **tablespoon chopped dill pickle**
1 **tablespoon reduced-calorie ketchup**
1 **teaspoon chopped fresh parsley**
⅛ **teaspoon salt**

STEPS IN PREPARATION:

1. Combine yogurt, buttermilk, and mayonnaise in a small bowl, stirring until blended. Stir in pickle and remaining ingredients.
2. Cover and chill.
3. Serve with salad greens.

Yield: ¾ cup

Note: See the Vegetable List on page 22 for exchange values of salad greens.

VINEGAR SALAD DRESSING

Exchanges: Free

Serving Size: 2 tablespoons
Carbohydrate: 4 gm
Protein: trace
Fat: trace

Calories: 15
Fiber: 0 gm
Sodium: 135 mg
Cholesterol: 0 mg

INGREDIENTS:

1 cup apple vinegar
2 tablespoons lemon juice
Sugar substitute to equal 4
  teaspoons sugar*
2 teaspoons finely chopped
  onion

1 teaspoon paprika
½ teaspoon salt
½ teaspoon dry mustard

STEPS IN PREPARATION:

1. Combine all ingredients in a jar; cover tightly, and shake vigorously. Chill.
2. Shake well before using.
3. Serve with salad greens.

Yield: 1 cup

Note: See the Vegetable List on page 22 for exchange values of salad greens.

*See the sugar substitution chart on page 354.

YOGURT-FRUIT SALAD DRESSING

Exchanges: Free

Serving Size: 2 tablespoons
Carbohydrate: 3 gm
Protein: 1 gm
Fat: trace

Calories: 17
Fiber: trace
Sodium: 233 mg
Cholesterol: trace

INGREDIENTS:

1 teaspoon grated orange rind
2 tablespoons unsweetened
   orange juice
2 tablespoons lemon juice

1 teaspoon salt
½ teaspoon dry mustard
¼ teaspoon paprika
1 cup plain low-fat yogurt

STEPS IN PREPARATION:

1. Combine first 6 ingredients in a small bowl, stirring until well blended; gently fold in yogurt.
2. Cover and chill.
3. Serve with fresh fruit salad.

Yield: 1¼ cups

Note: See the Fruit List on page 23 for exchange values of fruit.

ZERO SALAD DRESSING

Exchanges: Free

Serving Size: 2 tablespoons
Carbohydrate: 2 gm
Protein: trace
Fat: trace

Calories: 8
Fiber: 0 gm
Sodium: 178 mg
Cholesterol: 0 mg

INGREDIENTS:

½ cup tomato juice
2 tablespoons lemon juice or
   vinegar
1 tablespoon minced onion

⅛ teaspoon salt
⅛ teaspoon dried oregano
Dash of garlic powder
Dash of pepper

STEPS IN PREPARATION:

1. Combine all ingredients in a jar; cover tightly, and shake vigorously. Chill.
2. Shake well before using.
3. Serve with salad greens.

Yield: ½ cup

Note: See the Vegetable List on page 22 for exchange values of salad greens.

Sauces and Toppings

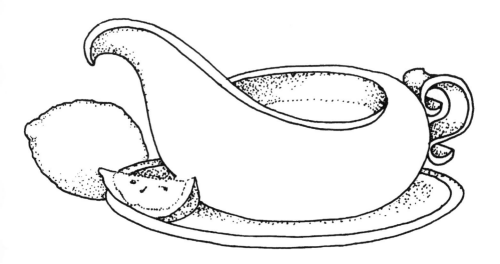

QUICK AND EASY BARBECUE SAUCE

Exchanges: Free

Serving Size: ½ cup
Carbohydrate: 3 gm
Protein: trace
Fat: trace

Calories: 13
Fiber: trace
Sodium: 148 mg
Cholesterol: 0 mg

INGREDIENTS:

2 cups sugar-free
cola-flavored carbonated
beverage

½ cup reduced-calorie
ketchup

STEPS IN PREPARATION:

1. Combine cola and ketchup, stirring until well blended.
2. Store in an airtight container in refrigerator.
3. Use as a marinating or basting sauce for meat or poultry.

Yield: 2½ cups

Note: See the Meat List on page 19 for exchange values of meat and poultry.

Basting lean meat and poultry with barbecue sauce
will help keep them from drying out as they cook
on the grill. Grilling is an easy way to add flavor
to food without adding fat. Coat the grill rack with
vegetable cooking spray to keep foods from sticking—it won't add many calories.

ZESTY BARBECUE SAUCE

Exchanges: Free

Serving Size: 2 tablespoons
Carbohydrate: 3 gm
Protein: trace
Fat: trace

Calories: 13
Fiber: 0 gm
Sodium: 135 mg
Cholesterol: 0 mg

INGREDIENTS:

½ cup lemon juice
⅓ cup cider vinegar
¼ cup cold water
¼ cup tomato juice
Sugar substitute to equal 4
  teaspoons sugar*
1 teaspoon dry mustard
1 teaspoon hot sauce

½ teaspoon salt
½ teaspoon onion powder
½ teaspoon paprika
½ teaspoon ground red
  pepper
½ teaspoon black pepper
⅛ teaspoon garlic powder
⅛ teaspoon dried oregano

STEPS IN PREPARATION:

1. Combine all ingredients in a medium saucepan. Bring mixture to a boil.
2. Transfer mixture to a serving container; cover and chill.
3. Serve with meat or poultry.

Yield: 1¼ cups

Note: See the Meat List on page 19 for exchange values of meat and poultry.

*See the sugar substitution chart on page 354.

CHEESE SAUCE

Exchanges: ½ Skim Milk, ½ Fat

Serving Size: ¼ cup	**Calories:** 78
Carbohydrate: 6 gm	**Fiber:** 0 gm
Protein: 6 gm	**Sodium:** 539 mg
Fat: 4 gm	**Cholesterol:** 9 mg

INGREDIENTS:

1 tablespoon all-purpose flour
1 cup skim milk, divided
1 tablespoon reduced-calorie margarine
½ cup (2 ounces) shredded low-fat process American cheese
½ teaspoon salt

STEPS IN PREPARATION:

1. Combine flour and ¼ cup milk; stir until smooth. Combine flour mixture, remaining ¾ cup milk, and margarine in a small saucepan; stir well. Cook over medium heat, stirring constantly, until mixture is thickened and bubbly.
2. Add shredded cheese and salt. Cook, stirring constantly, until cheese melts. (Do not overcook.)
3. Serve over vegetables.

Yield: 1 cup

Note: See the Vegetable List on page 22 for exchange values of vegetables.

COCKTAIL SAUCE

Exchanges: Free

Serving Size: 2 tablespoons
Carbohydrate: 4 gm
Protein: 1 gm
Fat: trace

Calories: 19
Fiber: 1 gm
Sodium: 459 mg
Cholesterol: 0 mg

INGREDIENTS:

½ cup tomato sauce
Sugar substitute to equal 2
  teaspoons sugar*
1 teaspoon finely chopped
  parsley
1 teaspoon lemon juice

½ teaspoon salt
½ teaspoon horseradish
½ teaspoon Worcestershire
  sauce
⅛ teaspoon dried oregano
Dash of onion powder

STEPS IN PREPARATION:

1. Combine all ingredients in a small bowl; stir well. Cover and chill.
2. Serve with baked, boiled, or broiled seafood.

Yield: ½ cup

Note: See the Meat List on page 19 for exchange values of seafood.

*See the sugar substitution chart on page 354.

FAT-FREE BEEF GRAVY

Exchanges: Free

Serving Size: 2 tablespoons	**Calories:** 5
Carbohydrate: 1 gm	**Fiber:** 0 gm
Protein: trace	**Sodium:** 76 mg
Fat: 0 gm	**Cholesterol:** 0 mg

INGREDIENTS:

2 tablespoons cornstarch or arrowroot

2 cups fat-free meat drippings or fat-free beef broth, divided

¼ teaspoon salt

¼ teaspoon pepper

½ cup minced onion (optional)

½ cup chopped mushrooms (optional)

2 tablespoons minced parsley (optional)

STEPS IN PREPARATION:

1. Add cornstarch to ½ cup broth, and stir.
2. Heat remaining 1½ cups broth in a saucepan. Add cornstarch mixture to hot broth. Add salt, pepper, and, if desired, onion, mushrooms, and parsley.
3. Reduce heat, and simmer, stirring constantly, until mixture thickens.

Yield: 3 cups

To make fat-free meat drippings, chill juices from cooked meats, and then skim off and discard fat. Use the fat-free juices for gravy or seasoning vegetables.

FAT-FREE CHICKEN GRAVY

Exchanges: Free

Serving Size: 2 tablespoons
Carbohydrate: 2 gm
Protein: 1 gm
Fat: trace

Calories: 15
Fiber: 0 gm
Sodium: 167 mg
Cholesterol: 0 mg

INGREDIENTS:

2 tablespoons all-purpose
   flour
¼ cup skim milk
1 cup fat-free chicken broth

½ teaspoon dried onion
   flakes
¼ teaspoon salt
¼ teaspoon pepper

STEPS IN PREPARATION:

1. Add flour to skim milk; stir until smooth.
2. Place broth and onion in a saucepan; bring to a boil.
3. Gradually add flour mixture to broth mixture, stirring constantly;
   stir in salt and pepper. Reduce heat; cook, stirring constantly, 5
   minutes.

Yield: 1 cup

Cornstarch and flour are two of the most common
thickening agents for sauces. Sauces that are thickened with flour look creamy; cornstarch-thickened
sauces appear more transparent.

GUACAMOLE

Exchanges: 1 Fat

Serving Size: 2 tablespoons	**Calories:** 50
Carbohydrate: 3 gm	**Fiber:** 1 gm
Protein: trace	**Sodium:** 166 mg
Fat: 4 gm	**Cholesterol:** 0 mg

INGREDIENTS:

2 large avocados, peeled, seeded, and mashed

3 canned green chiles, seeded and chopped

3 tablespoons lemon or lime juice

¼ teaspoon salt

STEPS IN PREPARATION:

1. Combine avocado and green chiles in a medium bowl, stirring to blend.
2. Add lemon juice and salt, stirring well. Cover and chill.
3. Serve with tortilla chips or as a topping for meat or poultry.

Yield: 1½ cups

Note: See the Starch List on page 16 for exchange values of chips and the Meat List on page 19 for exchange values of meat and poultry.

Serve red or blue corn tortilla chips with Guacamole for a festive look. The chips are made from naturally pigmented red and blue corn kernals. Red or blue chips can be found in specialty supermarkets and health food stores. Be sure to look for the low-salt, low-fat varieties.

GARDEN VEGETABLE MARINADE

Exchanges: Free

Serving Size: 2 tablespoons
Carbohydrate: 3 gm
Protein: trace
Fat: trace

Calories: 12
Fiber: trace
Sodium: 161 mg
Cholesterol: 0 mg

INGREDIENTS:

2 cups commercial no-oil
   Italian dressing
Sugar substitute to equal ¾
   cup sugar*

1 teaspoon salt
2 cloves garlic, crushed

STEPS IN PREPARATION:

1. Combine all ingredients in a jar. Cover tightly, and shake vigorously. Store in refrigerator.
2. Use as a marinade for fresh vegetables.

Yield: 2 cups

Note: See the Vegetable List on page 22 for exchange values of vegetables.

*See the sugar substitution chart on page 354.

SALSA

Exchanges: Free

Serving Size: 2 tablespoons	**Calories:** 16
Carbohydrate: 2 gm	**Fiber:** trace
Protein: trace	**Sodium:** 313 mg
Fat: trace	**Cholesterol:** 0 mg

INGREDIENTS:

2 medium tomatoes, peeled and chopped
3 tablespoons canned diced green chiles, drained

2 tablespoons minced onion
1 teaspoon vegetable oil
1 teaspoon vinegar
½ teaspoon salt

STEPS IN PREPARATION:

1. Combine all ingredients in a medium bowl, stirring well.
2. Transfer mixture to a serving container; cover and chill.
3. Serve with tortilla chips or as a topping for meat or poultry.

Yield: 1 cup

Note: See the Starch List on page 16 for exchange values of chips and the Meat List on page 19 for exchange values of meat and poultry.

Enjoy the convenience of low-fat snack products now available such as no-oil baked tortilla chips, fat-free potato chips, fat-free crackers, and baked rice snacks.

MEATLESS TOMATO SAUCE

Exchanges: 1 Vegetable

Serving Size: ½ cup
Carbohydrate: 6 gm
Protein: 1 gm
Fat: trace

Calories: 28
Fiber: 1 gm
Sodium: 452 mg
Cholesterol: 0 mg

INGREDIENTS:

1 (16-ounce) can no-salt-
   added whole tomatoes,
   undrained and chopped
1 tablespoon dried basil

1 teaspoon garlic powder
½ teaspoon salt
⅛ teaspoon pepper

STEPS IN PREPARATION:

1. Combine all ingredients in a medium saucepan, stirring until well blended.
2. Bring tomato mixture to a boil; reduce heat, and simmer, uncovered, 30 minutes, stirring occasionally.
3. Serve over cooked noodles (cooked without salt or fat).

Yield: 2 cups

Note: See the Starch List on page 16 for exchange value of noodles.

WHITE SAUCE

Exchanges: Free

Serving Size: 2 tablespoons	**Calories:** 20
Carbohydrate: 2 gm	**Fiber:** 0 gm
Protein: 1 gm	**Sodium:** 166 mg
Fat: 1 gm	**Cholesterol:** 1 mg

INGREDIENTS:

1 **tablespoon all-purpose flour**
1 **cup skim milk, divided**

1 **tablespoon reduced-calorie margarine**
½ **teaspoon salt**

STEPS IN PREPARATION:

1. Combine flour and ¼ cup milk; stir until smooth. Combine flour mixture, remaining ¾ cup milk, and margarine in a small saucepan; stir well. Cook over medium heat, stirring constantly, until mixture is thickened and bubbly.
2. Remove from heat, and stir in salt.
3. Serve with fish, meat, or poultry.

Yield: 1 cup

Note: See the Meat List on page 19 for exchange values of fish, meat, and poultry.

APPLE JELLY

Exchanges: Free

Serving Size: 1 tablespoon
Carbohydrate: 3 gm
Protein: trace
Fat: trace

Calories: 13
Fiber: 0 gm
Sodium: 1 mg
Cholesterol: 0 mg

INGREDIENTS:

1½ cups unsweetened apple
  juice
¾ teaspoon lemon juice
6 whole cloves
1 stick cinnamon

1½ teaspoons unflavored
  gelatin
⅓ cup cold water
Sugar substitute to equal ½
  cup sugar*

STEPS IN PREPARATION:

1. Combine first 4 ingredients in a heavy saucepan. Bring to a boil; reduce heat, and simmer 10 minutes.
2. Sprinkle gelatin over cold water; let stand 1 minute.
3. Remove juice mixture from heat; remove and discard cloves and cinnamon. Add gelatin mixture and sugar substitute, stirring until gelatin dissolves.
4. Pour carefully into 2 hot (8-ounce) jars. Cover lightly until cooled. Cover tightly, and store in refrigerator.
5. Serve with bread, toast, or crackers.

Yield: 1⅓ cups

Note: See the Starch List on page 16 for exchange values of bread, toast, and crackers.

*See the sugar substitution chart on page 354.

CRANBERRY SAUCE

Exchanges: Free

Serving Size: 2 tablespoons	**Calories:** 32
Carbohydrate: 8 gm	**Fiber:** 0 gm
Protein: trace	**Sodium:** 19 mg
Fat: trace	**Cholesterol:** 0 mg

INGREDIENTS:

Sugar substitute to equal 1
  cup sugar*
½ cup water
2 tablespoons grated
  orange rind
¼ teaspoon salt
⅛ teaspoon ground cinnamon
Dash of cloves
4 cups fresh ripe cranberries
½ teaspoon vanilla extract

STEPS IN PREPARATION:

1. Combine first 6 ingredients in a medium saucepan. Bring to a boil; reduce heat, and simmer 5 minutes, stirring occasionally.
2. Add cranberries; simmer 10 to 15 minutes or until skins pop. Remove from heat, and add vanilla. Cover and chill.
3. Serve with baked chicken or turkey.

Yield: 3¾ cups

Note: See the Meat List on page 19 for exchange values of chicken and turkey.

*See the sugar substitution chart on page 354.

STRAWBERRY SAUCE

Exchanges: Free

Serving Size: 1 tablespoon
Carbohydrate: 3 gm
Protein: trace
Fat: trace

Calories: 11
Fiber: trace
Sodium: 3 mg
Cholesterol: 0 mg

INGREDIENTS:

1 quart fresh strawberries, washed, hulled, and coarsely chopped
¾ cup cold water, divided
2 tablespoons lemon juice

¼ teaspoon ground cinnamon
3 tablespoons cornstarch
Sugar substitute to equal 1 cup sugar*

STEPS IN PREPARATION:

1. Combine strawberries, ½ cup water, lemon juice, and cinnamon in a small Dutch oven, stirring well; bring mixture to a boil.
2. Dissolve cornstarch in remaining ¼ cup water, and stir into strawberry mixture. Reduce heat, and simmer 2 to 3 minutes or until mixture thickens, stirring occasionally.
3. Remove from heat, and let cool. Stir in sugar substitute.
4. Serve with pancakes, waffles, or toast.

Yield: 2 cups

Note: See the Starch List on page 16 for exchange values of pancakes, waffles, and toast.

*See the sugar substitution chart on page 354.

WHIPPED TOPPING

Exchanges: Free

Serving Size: ¼ cup	**Calories:** 10
Carbohydrate: 2 gm	**Fiber:** 0 gm
Protein: trace	**Sodium:** 10 mg
Fat: trace	**Cholesterol:** trace

INGREDIENTS:

¼ cup ice water
¼ cup instant nonfat dry
   milk powder

Sugar substitute to equal ⅓
   cup sugar*
1 tablespoon lemon juice

STEPS IN PREPARATION:

1. Place ice water in a small bowl; gradually add milk powder, beating at high speed of an electric mixer until stiff peaks form.
2. Gently fold in sugar substitute and lemon juice. Cover and chill.
3. Use as a substitute for whipped cream.

Yield: 2½ cups

*See the sugar substitution chart on page 354.

Soups

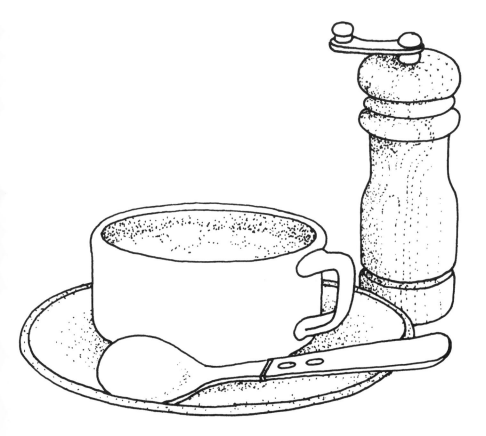

BROCCOLI-CAULIFLOWER SOUP

Exchanges: 1 Vegetable

Serving Size: ½ cup	**Calories:** 32
Carbohydrate: 5 gm	**Fiber:** 1 gm
Protein: 3 gm	**Sodium:** 274 mg
Fat: trace	**Cholesterol:** 1 mg

INGREDIENTS:

1½ cups water
1 (10-ounce) package frozen chopped broccoli, thawed
1 (10-ounce) package frozen cauliflower, thawed
⅓ cup chopped onion
2 teaspoons chicken-flavored bouillon granules
¼ teaspoon ground mace
1 tablespoon cornstarch
3 cups skim milk, divided
½ teaspoon salt
⅛ teaspoon pepper

STEPS IN PREPARATION:

1. Combine first 5 ingredients in a small Dutch oven. Cover and bring to a boil. Cook 5 to 8 minutes or until vegetables are tender (do not drain). Stir in mace.
2. Transfer vegetable mixture in batches to container of an electric blender or food processor; cover and process until smooth.
3. Return vegetable mixture to Dutch oven.
4. Dissolve cornstarch in ½ cup milk; stir into vegetable mixture.
5. Add remaining 2½ cups milk, salt, and pepper to vegetable mixture, stirring well.
6. Cook over medium heat until mixture is thickened and bubbly, stirring frequently.

Yield: 15 servings

FLAVORFUL ONION SOUP

Exchanges: 1 Vegetable

Serving Size: 2 cups
Carbohydrate: 3 gm
Protein: trace
Fat: 2 gm

Calories: 24
Fiber: trace
Sodium: 45 mg
Cholesterol: 0 mg

INGREDIENTS:

1 tablespoon reduced-calorie margarine
1 medium onion, thinly sliced
5½ cups water
1 tablespoon plus 2 teaspoons low-sodium beef-flavored bouillon granules

½ teaspoon Worcestershire sauce

STEPS IN PREPARATION:

1. Melt margarine in a medium saucepan over low heat; add onion. Cover and cook over low heat 20 minutes or until onion is lightly browned, stirring occasionally.
2. Add water, bouillon granules, and Worcestershire sauce, stirring well.
3. Cover and bring to a boil. Reduce heat, and simmer 10 minutes.

Yield: 3 servings

ENGLISH PEA SOUP

Exchanges: ½ Starch

Serving Size: ½ cup	**Calories:** 45
Carbohydrate: 8 gm	**Fiber:** 3 gm
Protein: 3 gm	**Sodium:** 372 mg
Fat: trace	**Cholesterol:** trace

INGREDIENTS:

1 (10-ounce) package frozen
  English peas
¼ medium head lettuce
3 ounces fresh spinach
½ cup chopped green onions
2 teaspoons chicken-flavored
  bouillon granules

½ teaspoon dried chervil,
  crushed
⅛ teaspoon pepper
1¼ cups water
¾ cup skim milk

STEPS IN PREPARATION:

1. Combine first 7 ingredients in a medium saucepan; stir in water. Cover and bring to a boil; reduce heat, and simmer 20 minutes.
2. Transfer mixture to container of an electric blender or food processor; cover and process until smooth.
3. Return mixture to saucepan; stir in milk.
4. Cook over medium heat until thoroughly heated, stirring frequently.

Yield: 8 servings

CREAMED POTATO SOUP

Exchanges: 1 Starch

Serving Size: ¾ cup
Carbohydrate: 14 gm
Protein: 2 gm
Fat: trace

Calories: 65
Fiber: 1 gm
Sodium: 144 mg
Cholesterol: trace

INGREDIENTS:

4 medium round red
   potatoes, peeled and sliced
1 small onion, peeled and
   sliced
4 green onions, coarsely
   chopped
2 (10½-ounce) cans no-salt-
   added chicken broth,
   undiluted

1 clove garlic, minced
1 cup skim milk
½ teaspoon salt
⅛ teaspoon ground white
   pepper
⅛ teaspoon ground nutmeg

STEPS IN PREPARATION:

1. Combine first 5 ingredients in a heavy 3-quart saucepan. Cover and simmer 20 minutes or until potato is tender.
2. Transfer potato mixture in batches to container of an electric blender or food processor; cover and process until smooth.
3. Combine pureed mixture with milk and remaining ingredients, stirring until well blended. Serve warm or chilled.

Yield: 9 servings

Reduce calories, fat, and cholesterol in cream-based soups by using skim milk in place of whipping cream or half-and-half.

TOMATO BOUILLON

Exchanges: 1 Vegetable

Serving Size: ¾ cup
Carbohydrate: 4 gm
Protein: 1 gm
Fat: trace

Calories: 17
Fiber: 1 gm
Sodium: 343 mg
Cholesterol: 0 mg

INGREDIENTS:

1¾ cups water
1½ cups tomato juice
2 teaspoons low-sodium
  beef-flavored bouillon
  granules

1 teaspoon Worcestershire
  sauce
⅛ teaspoon hot sauce

STEPS IN PREPARATION:

1. Combine all ingredients in a medium saucepan, stirring until bouillon granules dissolve.
2. Cover and bring to a boil. Reduce heat, and simmer 10 minutes.

Yield: 4 servings

No-salt-added tomato juice will make this recipe lower in sodium.

VEGETABLE-CHEESE SOUP

Exchanges: 1 Vegetable, ½ Skim Milk

Serving Size: 1 cup	**Calories:** 71
Carbohydrate: 12 gm	**Fiber:** 2 gm
Protein: 4 gm	**Sodium:** 384 mg
Fat: 1 gm	**Cholesterol:** 3 mg

INGREDIENTS:

1 (10-ounce) package frozen mixed vegetables, thawed
1 small onion, diced
2 tablespoons all-purpose flour
1 teaspoon dried Italian seasoning
¼ teaspoon salt
⅛ teaspoon pepper
1 cup water
1 cup skim milk
1 teaspoon chicken-flavored bouillon granules
¼ cup (1 ounce) shredded low-fat process American cheese
2 teaspoons Dijon mustard

STEPS IN PREPARATION:

1. Combine mixed vegetables and onion in a medium saucepan.
2. Combine flour, Italian seasoning, salt, and pepper, stirring well; add to vegetables, and stir to coat.
3. Combine water and milk; add bouillon granules, stirring until granules dissolve. Add to vegetable mixture, and bring to a boil.
4. Cook, stirring constantly, 5 minutes or until mixture is thickened and bubbly.
5. Reduce heat to low; add cheese and mustard, stirring to blend. Serve immediately.

Yield: 6 servings

ZUCCHINI SOUP

Exchanges: 1 Starch

Serving Size: 1 cup	**Calories:** 108
Carbohydrate: 22 gm	**Fiber:** 4 gm
Protein: 4 gm	**Sodium:** 65 mg
Fat: 2 gm	**Cholesterol:** trace

INGREDIENTS:

5 cups chopped zucchini
1 large baking potato, peeled
   and cut into 1-inch cubes
1 cup water
3 green onions, thinly sliced
1 tablespoon reduced-calorie
   margarine, melted

½ cup water
1½ teaspoons dried tarragon
½ teaspoon chicken-flavored
   bouillon granules
½ cup skim milk

STEPS IN PREPARATION:

1. Combine zucchini, potato, and 1 cup water in a small Dutch oven. Cover and bring to a boil. Boil 10 minutes or until crisp-tender (do not drain).
2. Sauté onions in margarine in a nonstick skillet until tender; add to zucchini mixture. Add ½ cup water, tarragon, and bouillon granules, stirring to blend.
3. Add skim milk, and cook over medium heat until thoroughly heated, stirring frequently.

Yield: 4 servings

QUICK BEEF SOUP

Exchanges: 1 Medium-Fat Meat, 1½ Vegetable

Serving Size: ½ cup	**Calories:** 98
Carbohydrate: 9 gm	**Fiber:** 2 gm
Protein: 7 gm	**Sodium:** 420 mg
Fat: 4 gm	**Cholesterol:** 16 mg

INGREDIENTS:

½ pound ground chuck
2 cups sliced carrot
¼ cup chopped onion
2 (8-ounce) cans tomato
   sauce
1 (2½-ounce) jar sliced
   mushrooms, drained
2 cups water

STEPS IN PREPARATION:

1. Cook ground chuck in a large nonstick skillet over medium heat until browned, stirring until meat crumbles. Drain and pat dry with paper towels. Wipe pan drippings from skillet with a paper towel.
2. Return meat to skillet; add carrot, onion, tomato sauce, and mushrooms. Stir in water.
3. Cover and bring to a boil. Reduce heat, and simmer 30 to 35 minutes or until carrot is tender, stirring occasionally.

Yield: 8 servings

GARDEN CHICKEN SOUP

Exchanges: 1 Starch, ½ Lean Meat

Serving Size: 1 cup	**Calories:** 101
Carbohydrate: 16 gm	**Fiber:** 2 gm
Protein: 6 gm	**Sodium:** 267 mg
Fat: 1 gm	**Cholesterol:** 8 mg

INGREDIENTS:

6 cups water
2 cups tomato juice
1 cup peeled, diced potato
1 cup chopped onion
1 cup whole kernel corn
1 cup cooked, drained lima beans
¾ cup chopped cooked chicken breast (skinned before cooking and cooked without salt)

½ cup sliced carrot
½ cup chopped celery
2 tablespoons low-sodium chicken-flavored bouillon granules
1 teaspoon garlic powder
1½ teaspoons Worcestershire sauce

STEPS IN PREPARATION:

1. Combine all ingredients in a large Dutch oven. Cover and bring to a boil.
2. Reduce heat, and simmer 45 minutes.

Yield: 10 servings

> Simple garnishes such as a sprinkling of fresh herbs or green onions, a slice of lemon, or a teaspoon of nonfat sour cream give soups an added touch of flavor and color.

NAVY BEAN SOUP

Exchanges: 2 Starch

Serving Size: 1 cup	**Calories:** 160
Carbohydrate: 30 gm	**Fiber:** 8 gm
Protein: 9 gm	**Sodium:** 283 mg
Fat: 1 gm	**Cholesterol:** 0 mg

INGREDIENTS:

1 (16-ounce) package dried navy beans
2 quarts water
1½ cups diced onion
¼ cup diced celery
1 tablespoon reduced-calorie margarine, melted
2 cups canned stewed tomatoes, drained
1 teaspoon salt

STEPS IN PREPARATION:

1. Sort and wash beans; place in a large Dutch oven. Cover with water 2 inches above beans; soak overnight. Drain beans.
2. Combine beans and 2 quarts water; bring to a boil. Cover, reduce heat, and simmer 2 hours.
3. Sauté onion and celery in margarine until tender; add onion mixture, tomato, and salt to bean mixture, stirring well.
4. Simmer, uncovered, 1 hour or until beans are tender.

Yield: 11 servings

COUNTRY CHILI

Exchanges: 1 Starch

Serving Size: ⅔ cup	**Calories:** 85
Carbohydrate: 15 gm	**Fiber:** 4 gm
Protein: 4 gm	**Sodium:** 598 mg
Fat: 1 gm	**Cholesterol:** 0 mg

INGREDIENTS:

1 large onion, chopped
1 clove garlic, chopped
1 tablespoon reduced-calorie margarine, melted
1 teaspoon salt
1 teaspoon dried basil
1 teaspoon chili powder
½ teaspoon dried oregano

½ teaspoon dried thyme
¼ teaspoon pepper
1 (16-ounce) can whole tomatoes, undrained and chopped
1 (8-ounce) can red kidney beans, undrained

STEPS IN PREPARATION:

1. Sauté onion and garlic in margarine in a large saucepan until tender.
2. Add salt and next 5 ingredients, stirring well.
3. Stir in tomato and beans. Simmer, uncovered, 10 to 15 minutes or until thoroughly heated.

Yield: 6 servings

Kidney beans are legumes, a class of vegetables that also includes pinto beans and other dried peas and beans. They're an especially good source of protein, are packed with fiber, and have no saturated fat or cholesterol. A ½-cup serving of red kidney beans provides as much iron as 6 ounces of lean red meat but only a trace of the fat.

Desserts

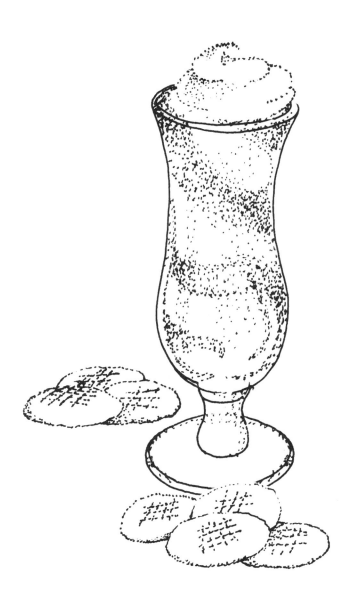

AMBROSIA

Exchanges: 1 Fruit, ½ Fat

Serving Size: ½ cup	**Calories:** 86
Carbohydrate: 15 gm	**Fiber:** 2 gm
Protein: 1 gm	**Sodium:** 2 mg
Fat: 3 gm	**Cholesterol:** 0 mg

INGREDIENTS:

2 medium oranges, peeled
1 small banana, peeled
20 seedless green grapes,
    halved

¼ cup unsweetened shredded
    coconut

STEPS IN PREPARATION:

1. Section oranges, and cut into small pieces.
2. Cut banana into thin slices.
3. Combine orange slices, banana, grape halves, and coconut. Cover and chill.

Yield: 5 servings

Be sure to purchase unsweetened shredded coconut–¼ cup of unsweetened coconut contains about 5 grams of carbohydrate; ¼ cup of sweetened coconut contains 44 grams of carbohydrate.

SPICED FRUIT

Exchanges: 1 Fruit

Serving Size: ½ cup	**Calories:** 91
Carbohydrate: 17 gm	**Fiber:** 4 gm
Protein: 1 gm	**Sodium:** 2 mg
Fat: trace	**Cholesterol:** 0 mg

INGREDIENTS:

1 medium orange
1 (15¼-ounce) can pineapple
  chunks in juice
2 (16-ounce) cans pear halves
  in juice, drained

1 (16-ounce) can apricot
  halves in juice, drained
6 whole cloves
2 (2-inch) sticks cinnamon

STEPS IN PREPARATION:

1. Peel orange, reserving rind. Section orange; remove and discard seeds.
2. Drain pineapple, reserving juice.
3. Combine orange, pineapple, pear, and apricot in a large bowl; set aside.
4. Combine orange rind, reserved pineapple juice, cloves, and cinnamon in a small saucepan, stirring well. Bring to a boil; reduce heat, and simmer 5 minutes. Remove from heat.
5. Strain juice mixture, discarding rind and whole spices. Pour juice over fruit, tossing gently to combine. Cover and chill.

Yield: 12 servings

BAKED APPLES

Exchanges: 1 Fruit

Serving Size: 1 apple	**Calories:** 98
Carbohydrate: 24 gm	**Fiber:** 2 gm
Protein: 1 gm	**Sodium:** 2 mg
Fat: trace	**Cholesterol:** 0 mg

INGREDIENTS:

4 small cooking apples
1 cup water
Sugar substitute to equal 8
  teaspoons sugar*

1 tablespoon lemon juice
½ teaspoon ground cinnamon
½ teaspoon ground nutmeg

STEPS IN PREPARATION:

1. Wash and core apples; cut a small slice from the top and bottom of each apple. Place apples in a small baking dish.
2. Combine water and remaining ingredients; pour over apples. Bake at 350° for 45 minutes or until tender, basting every 15 minutes.

Yield: 4 servings

*See the sugar substitution chart on page 354.

Some of the best cooking apple varieties are Baldwin, Cortland, Granny Smith, Northern Spy, Rome Beauty, Winesap, and York Imperial.

SUGARLESS APPLE DESSERT

Exchanges: 2 Fruit

Serving Size: ½ cup
Carbohydrate: 35 gm
Protein: 4 gm
Fat: 1 gm

Calories: 166
Fiber: 1 gm
Sodium: 44 mg
Cholesterol: 0 mg

INGREDIENTS:

3 envelopes unflavored gelatin
1 (12-ounce) can unsweetened frozen apple juice concentrate, diluted with 1 can water

1 teaspoon ground cinnamon
½ teaspoon ground nutmeg
5 cups peeled, sliced apple
1 tablespoon reduced-calorie margarine

STEPS IN PREPARATION:

1. Combine first 4 ingredients in a large skillet, stirring well; let stand 1 minute. Cook over low heat 1 minute or until gelatin dissolves.
2. Add apple. Cover and cook over low heat 20 to 25 minutes or until tender, stirring frequently.
3. Add margarine; stir gently until margarine melts. Remove from heat. Cover and chill.
4. To serve, spoon mixture evenly into individual dessert dishes.

Yield: 5 servings

SPICED BAKED BANANAS

Exchanges: 1 Fruit

Serving Size: ½ banana
Carbohydrate: 11 gm
Protein: trace
Fat: trace

Calories: 43
Fiber: 1 gm
Sodium: 9 mg
Cholesterol: 0 mg

INGREDIENTS:

3 small, very ripe bananas, peeled
Vegetable cooking spray
4 teaspoons granulated brown sugar substitute

2 teaspoons grated lemon rind
½ teaspoon vanilla extract
⅛ teaspoon ground cinnamon

STEPS IN PREPARATION:

1. Cut bananas in half lenthwise; place bananas in an 11- x 7- x 2-inch baking dish coated with cooking spray.
2. Sprinkle with brown sugar substitute and remaining ingredients. Bake at 350° for 15 to 20 minutes or until thoroughly heated. Serve warm.

Yield: 6 servings

Keep ripe bananas an extra three to five days by refrigerating them. Or peel, mash, and freeze bananas, and store in airtight containers to use in baking. Even if bananas are past their prime, you can remove any brown portions and puree the rest to make banana bread, banana cake, or banana muffins.

BRANDIED ORANGES

Exchanges: 1 Fruit

Serving Size: ¼ cup
Carbohydrate: 18 gm
Protein: 1 gm
Fat: trace

Calories: 50
Fiber: 2 gm
Sodium: 2 mg
Cholesterol: 0 mg

INGREDIENTS:

3 large oranges, peeled and
   sectioned
⅓ cup raisins
¼ cup unsweetened orange
   juice

1 teaspoon brandy extract
¼ cup slivered almonds,
   toasted

STEPS IN PREPARATION:

1. Place orange sections in a medium bowl. Combine raisins, orange juice, and brandy extract; add to orange sections. Cover and chill overnight, stirring occasionally.
2. Sprinkle with almonds before serving.

Yield: 12 servings

CINNAMON ORANGES

Exchanges: 1 Fruit

Serving Size: ½ cup
Carbohydrate: 18 gm
Protein: 1 gm
Fat: trace

Calories: 73
Fiber: 3 gm
Sodium: 2 mg
Cholesterol: 0 mg

INGREDIENTS:

Sugar substitute to equal ¼
  cup sugar*
¾ teaspoon ground cinnamon
¼ teaspoon ground cloves

4 medium oranges, peeled
  and thinly sliced
¼ cup water
½ teaspoon rum extract

STEPS IN PREPARATION:

1. Combine sugar substitute, cinnamon, and cloves in a small bowl.
2. Arrange half of orange slices in a 1-quart bowl; sprinkle with half of cinnamon mixture. Add remaining orange slices and remaining cinnamon mixture.
3. Combine water and rum extract; pour over orange mixture. Cover and chill overnight.
4. Spoon juice over oranges to moisten before serving.

Yield: 4 servings

*See the sugar substitution chart on page 354.

ORANGE DELIGHT

Exchanges: 1 Skim Milk

Serving Size: ¾ cup
Carbohydrate: 14 gm
Protein: 8 gm
Fat: trace

Calories: 95
Fiber: 1 gm
Sodium: 267 mg
Cholesterol: 3 mg

INGREDIENTS:

Whipped Topping (page 302)
2 cups 1% low-fat cottage
  cheese
2 (15¼-ounce) cans crushed
  pineapple in juice, well
  drained

1 (0.3-ounce) package sugar-
  free orange-flavored gelatin
Fresh mint sprigs (optional)

STEPS IN PREPARATION:

1. Spoon Whipped Topping into a medium bowl. Gently fold in
   cottage cheese, pineapple, and gelatin.
2. Spoon mixture evenly into individual dessert dishes, and garnish
   each serving with mint sprigs, if desired.

Yield: 8 servings

BAKED SPICED PEARS

Exchanges: 1 Fruit

Serving Size: ½ cup	**Calories:** 56
Carbohydrate: 13 gm	**Fiber:** 3 gm
Protein: trace	**Sodium:** 44 mg
Fat: 1 gm	**Cholesterol:** 0 mg

INGREDIENTS:

6 medium pears, peeled and sliced
¾ cup granulated brown sugar substitute
2 tablespoons crystallized ginger

1½ teaspoons rum extract
¼ teaspoon ground cinnamon
Dash of ground allspice
2 teaspoons reduced-calorie margarine

STEPS IN PREPARATION:

1. Arrange pear slices in an 11- x 7- x 2-inch baking dish.
2. Combine brown sugar substitute, ginger, rum extract, cinnamon, and allspice.
3. Sprinkle brown sugar mixture over pears; dot with margarine. Bake at 350° for 20 minutes. Serve warm or chilled.

Yield: 12 servings

Crystallized ginger is ginger that has been cooked in a sugar syrup and coated with coarse sugar. The amount of sugar in 2 tablespoons crystallized ginger has been calculated into this recipe and is acceptable for use in the diet plans of most people with diabetes.

PEACH CRUMB BAKE

Exchanges: 1 Fruit, ½ Fat

Serving Size: ½ cup	**Calories:** 75
Carbohydrate: 15 gm	**Fiber:** 2 gm
Protein: 1 gm	**Sodium:** 68 mg
Fat: 2 gm	**Cholesterol:** trace

INGREDIENTS:

2 cups sliced fresh peaches
Vegetable cooking spray
⅓ cup graham cracker
  crumbs

½ teaspoon ground cinnamon
⅛ teaspoon ground nutmeg
2 teaspoons reduced-calorie
  margarine, melted

STEPS IN PREPARATION:

1. Arrange peach slices in bottom of an 8-inch square baking dish coated with cooking spray.
2. Combine graham cracker crumbs, cinnamon, and nutmeg in a small bowl, stirring well. Add margarine, and stir until blended.
3. Sprinkle graham cracker crumb mixture over peaches, and bake at 350° for 30 minutes. Serve warm.

Yield: 4 servings

PINEAPPLE DESSERT

Exchanges: 1 Fruit

Serving Size: ½ cup	**Calories:** 70
Carbohydrate: 15 gm	**Fiber:** 1 gm
Protein: 3 gm	**Sodium:** 35 mg
Fat: trace	**Cholesterol:** 1 mg

INGREDIENTS:

1 (15¼-ounce) can crushed pineapple in juice
1 envelope unflavored gelatin
¼ teaspoon vanilla extract
½ cup instant nonfat dry milk powder
⅓ cup ice water
2 tablespoons lemon juice
Sugar substitute to equal 2 teaspoons sugar*

STEPS IN PREPARATION:

1. Drain pineapple, reserving juice. Set pineapple aside. Add water, if necessary, to pineapple juice to yield 1 cup.
2. Combine juice mixture and gelatin in a small saucepan, stirring well; let stand 1 minute. Cook over low heat, stirring constantly, 1 minute or until gelatin dissolves. Remove from heat, and stir in pineapple and vanilla. Cover and chill until mixture reaches the consistency of unbeaten egg white.
3. Combine milk powder and ice water in a medium bowl; beat at medium speed of an electric mixer until foamy. Add lemon juice; beat 3 to 4 minutes or until stiff peaks form, gradually adding sugar substitute.
4. Fold gelatin mixture into whipped milk mixture. Spoon evenly into 6 (6-ounce) custard cups or dessert dishes. Cover and chill.

Yield: 6 servings

*See the sugar substitution chart on page 354.

FRUIT MELBA

Exchanges: 1 Fruit

Serving Size: ¾ cup	**Calories:** 59
Carbohydrate: 14 gm	**Fiber:** 2 gm
Protein: 1 gm	**Sodium:** 11 mg
Fat: trace	**Cholesterol:** 0 mg

INGREDIENTS:

½ cup reduced-calorie
   cranberry juice
1 teaspoon cornstarch
4 drops almond extract

1 cup fresh or frozen
   unsweetened raspberries
3 cups cantaloupe balls

STEPS IN PREPARATION:

1. Combine cranberry juice and cornstarch in a small saucepan. Cook over medium heat, stirring constantly, until mixture is thick and bubbly.
2. Remove cranberry juice mixture from heat; stir in almond extract, and let cool.
3. Combine raspberries and cantaloupe balls; spoon ½ cup fruit mixture into each of 4 dessert dishes. Top evenly with cranberry juice mixture.

Yield: 4 servings

Featuring fruit as the main ingredient in desserts offers several nutritional benefits. Thanks to the natural sweetness of most fruit, you don't need to add much (if any) sugar. Fruit desserts also provide more vitamin, more fiber, and fewer calories than other types of desserts.

BAKED CUSTARD

Exchanges: ½ Skim Milk, ½ Fat

Serving Size: ½ cup
Carbohydrate: 8 gm
Protein: 6 gm
Fat: 2 gm

Calories: 76
Fiber: 0 gm
Sodium: 73 mg
Cholesterol: 77 mg

INGREDIENTS:

2 eggs
2 cups skim milk
Liquid sugar substitute to
 equal ⅓ cup sugar*

2 teaspoons vanilla extract

STEPS IN PREPARATION:

1. Lightly beat eggs in a small bowl; add milk, sugar substitute, and vanilla, and beat well.
2. Pour mixture evenly into 5 (6-ounce) custard cups, and place cups in a baking pan containing 1 inch hot water. Bake at 350° for 45 minutes or until a knife inserted in center comes out clean. Cover and chill thoroughly.

Yield: 5 servings

*See the sugar substitution chart on page 354.

Baked puddings thickened with eggs are often cooked in a baking pan filled with about 1 inch of water. The gentle heat from this cooking method helps to keep the pudding from breaking or curdling during cooking.

PUMPKIN CUSTARD

Exchanges: ½ Starch, ½ Medium-Fat Meat

Serving Size: ½ cup
Carbohydrate: 10 gm
Protein: 5 gm
Fat: 2 gm

Calories: 72
Fiber: 1 gm
Sodium: 98 mg
Cholesterol: 63 mg

INGREDIENTS:

1½ cups canned pumpkin
1½ cups skim milk
Sugar substitute to equal 2
 tablespoons sugar*
¾ teaspoon ground
 cinnamon
¼ teaspoon ground allspice
¼ teaspoon ground cloves
¼ teaspoon ground ginger
¼ teaspoon ground nutmeg
⅛ teaspoon salt
2 eggs, well beaten

STEPS IN PREPARATION:

1. Combine all ingredients, and stir well.
2. Pour mixture evenly into 6 (6-ounce) custard cups. Set cups in a baking pan containing 1 inch hot water.
3. Bake at 425° for 10 minutes. Reduce heat to 350°, and bake for 20 minutes or until a knife inserted in center comes out clean. Serve warm or chilled.

Yield: 6 servings

*See the sugar substitution chart on page 354.

CHOCOLATE AND FRUIT PARFAITS

Exchanges: 1 Fruit, ½ Skim Milk

Serving Size: 1 parfait	**Calories:** 118
Carbohydrate: 24 gm	**Fiber:** 2 gm
Protein: 5 gm	**Sodium:** 90 mg
Fat: trace	**Cholesterol:** 2 mg

INGREDIENTS:

1 cup cold water
2 tablespoons unsweetened cocoa
Sugar substitute to equal ½ cup plus 2 tablespoons sugar, divided*

1 cup instant nonfat dry milk powder
2 cups sliced fresh strawberries, divided
2 medium bananas, peeled and sliced

STEPS IN PREPARATION:

1. Combine water and cocoa in a small saucepan; bring to a boil, stirring constantly with a wire whisk to dissolve cocoa. Remove from heat, and let cool. Stir in half of sugar substitute. Cover and chill.
2. Add milk powder to cocoa mixture, and beat at high speed of an electric mixer until mixture is thick and fluffy. Cover and chill.
3. Sprinkle remaining half of sugar substitute over strawberries; let stand at room temperature 20 minutes. Place half of sliced strawberries evenly in 6 parfait glasses. Set remaining strawberries aside.
4. Spoon chilled cocoa mixture evenly over strawberries in parfait glasses; arrange banana slices evenly over top. Top parfaits evenly with remaining strawberries.

Yield: 6 servings

*See the sugar substitution chart on page 354.

BERRY PUDDING

Exchanges: 1 Fruit

Serving Size: ½ cup
Carbohydrate: 17 gm
Protein: 1 gm
Fat: trace

Calories: 70
Fiber: 1 gm
Sodium: 46 mg
Cholesterol: 0 mg

INGREDIENTS:

3 cups fresh or frozen
  unsweetened berries,
  divided
1 cup water
3 tablespoons cornstarch
⅛ teaspoon salt

⅛ teaspoon ground
  cinnamon
Sugar substitute to equal 1
  cup sugar*
½ teaspoon vanilla or almond
  extract

STEPS IN PREPARATION:

1. Combine 1 cup berries, water, cornstarch, salt, and cinnamon in a
   medium saucepan. Cook over medium heat, stirring constantly,
   until mixture thickens.
2. Add remaining 2 cups berries, sugar substitute, and vanilla; stir
   well. Let cool before serving.

Yield: 6 servings

Note: Serve with Whipped Topping (page 302), if desired.

*See the sugar substitution chart on page 354.

OLD-FASHIONED BREAD PUDDING

Exchanges: 2 Starch, 1 Fat

Serving Size: ½ cup	**Calories:** 166
Carbohydrate: 25 gm	**Fiber:** 1 gm
Protein: 7 gm	**Sodium:** 191 mg
Fat: 4 gm	**Cholesterol:** 95 mg

INGREDIENTS:

6 slices white bread, crusts removed
2 tablespoons reduced-calorie margarine, melted
Sugar substitute to equal ¾ cup sugar, divided*
1 teaspoon ground cinnamon
½ cup raisins
Vegetable cooking spray
4 eggs, lightly beaten
2 cups skim milk
1 teaspoon vanilla extract

STEPS IN PREPARATION:

1. Brush bread lightly with melted margarine; sprinkle evenly with one-third of the sugar substitute and cinnamon.
2. Cut bread slices into quarters. Layer bread and raisins in a 1½-quart casserole coated with cooking spray.
3. Combine eggs, milk, vanilla, and remaining two-thirds of sugar substitute; pour over bread and raisins in dish.
4. Place dish in a baking pan containing 1 inch hot water. Bake at 350° for 55 minutes to 1 hour or until a knife inserted in center comes out clean. Serve warm or chilled.

Yield: 8 servings

*See the sugar substitution chart on page 354.

BAKED LEMON PUDDING

Exchanges: 1 Lowfat Milk

Serving Size: ½ cup	**Calories:** 114
Carbohydrate: 13 gm	**Fiber:** 0 gm
Protein: 6 gm	**Sodium:** 199 mg
Fat: 4 gm	**Cholesterol:** 95 mg

INGREDIENTS:

3 eggs, separated
Sugar substitute to equal ½ cup sugar*
¼ teaspoon salt
1½ cups skim milk
¼ cup plus 1 tablespoon all-purpose flour
¼ teaspoon grated lemon rind
⅓ cup plus 1 tablespoon lemon juice
2 tablespoons reduced-calorie margarine, melted

STEPS IN PREPARATION:

1. Combine egg whites, sugar substitute, and salt; beat at high speed of an electric mixer until soft peaks form.
2. Combine egg yolks, milk, and remaining ingredients; beat until smooth. Fold in egg white mixture.
3. Pour mixture evenly into 6 (6-ounce) custard cups. Place custard cups in a baking pan containing 1 inch hot water. Cover and bake at 325° for 1 hour or until a knife inserted in center comes out clean.

Yield: 6 servings

*See the sugar substitution chart on page 354.

TAPIOCA PUDDING

Exchanges: ½ Skim Milk

Serving Size: ⅓ cup
Carbohydrate: 9 gm
Protein: 3 gm
Fat: trace

Calories: 57
Fiber: 0 gm
Sodium: 46 mg
Cholesterol: 33 mg

INGREDIENTS:

1 egg, separated
1¾ cups skim milk
3 tablespoons tapioca
Sugar substitute to equal 2
   tablespoons sugar*

½ teaspoon vanilla extract
1 drop yellow food coloring

STEPS IN PREPARATION:

1. Combine egg yolk, milk, tapioca, and sugar substitute in a medium saucepan. Cook over low heat, stirring constantly, until mixture comes to a boil. Remove from heat, and let cool.
2. Add vanilla and food coloring.
3. Beat egg white at high speed of an electric mixer until stiff peaks form; fold into tapioca mixture. Spoon evenly into individual dessert dishes.

Yield: 6 servings

*See the sugar substitution chart on page 354.

STRAWBERRY MOUSSE

Exchanges: ½ Skim Milk

Serving Size: ½ cup
Carbohydrate: 7 gm
Protein: 4 gm
Fat: trace

Calories: 45
Fiber: trace
Sodium: 78 mg
Cholesterol: 1 mg

INGREDIENTS:

1 (0.3-ounce) package sugar-free strawberry-flavored gelatin
½ cup water
1½ cups sliced fresh strawberries
⅔ cup instant nonfat dry milk powder
6 ice cubes

STEPS IN PREPARATION:

1. Combine gelatin and water in a small saucepan, stirring well; let stand 1 minute. Cook over low heat, stirring constantly, 1 minute or until gelatin dissolves.
2. Combine gelatin mixture, strawberries, and milk powder in container of an electric blender; cover and process until smooth. Add ice cubes, one at a time, processing until blended.
3. Spoon mixture evenly into 6 parfait glasses. Cover and chill.

Yield: 6 servings

HOMESTYLE APPLE PIE

Exchanges: ½ Starch, 1 Fruit, ½ Fat

Serving Size: ⅛ pie	**Calories:** 126
Carbohydrate: 23 gm	**Fiber:** 2 gm
Protein: 2 gm	**Sodium:** 338 mg
Fat: 3 gm	**Cholesterol:** 0 mg

INGREDIENTS:

Sugar substitute to equal ⅓ cup sugar*
1 tablespoon cornstarch
½ teaspoon grated lemon rind
1 teaspoon lemon juice
½ teaspoon ground cinnamon
¼ teaspoon ground nutmeg
4 small apples, peeled and sliced
1 cup all-purpose flour
1 teaspoon salt
¼ cup reduced-calorie margarine
3 tablespoons cold water

STEPS IN PREPARATION:

1. Combine first 7 ingredients. Place in a 9-inch deep-dish pieplate; set aside.
2. Combine flour and salt; cut in margarine with a pastry blender until mixture resembles coarse meal. Add water, stirring with a fork until dry ingredients are moistened.
3. Shape dough into a ball; roll out on a floured surface, and place on top of apple filling. Bake at 425° for 30 minutes or until lightly browned.

Yield: 8 servings

*See the sugar substitution chart on page 354.

APPLESAUCE-SPICE BUNDT CAKE

Exchanges: 1 Starch, 1 Fruit, 2 Fat

Serving Size: 1 slice	**Calories:** 204
Carbohydrate: 28 gm	**Fiber:** 2 gm
Protein: 3 gm	**Sodium:** 287 mg
Fat: 9 gm	**Cholesterol:** 22 mg

INGREDIENTS:

1 cup water
1½ cups golden raisins
3 tablespoons self-rising flour
2 cups unsweetened
  applesauce
2 eggs, lightly beaten
Sugar substitute to equal
  ¾ cup sugar*

¾ cup vegetable oil
2 tablespoons vanilla extract
3 cups self-rising flour
¼ teaspoon baking soda
2 teaspoons ground cinnamon
½ teaspoon ground allspice
Vegetable cooking spray

STEPS IN PREPARATION:

1. Combine 1 cup water and raisins in a medium saucepan; bring to a boil. Boil until water is completely absorbed; remove from heat. Add 3 tablespoons flour; toss well.
2. Combine applesauce and next 4 ingredients; stir well. Combine 3 cups flour and next 3 ingredients. Gradually add to applesauce mixture, stirring just until dry ingredients are moistened. Fold in raisins.
3. Pour batter into a 10-inch Bundt pan coated with cooking spray. Bake at 350° for 45 minutes or until a wooden pick inserted in center comes out clean. Cool in pan 10 minutes; remove from pan, and cool completely on a wire rack.

Yield: 20 servings

*See the sugar substitution chart on page 354.

CHEESECAKE

Exchanges: ½ Starch, 1 Lowfat Milk

Serving Size: 1 slice	**Calories:** 135
Carbohydrate: 19 gm	**Fiber:** 1 gm
Protein: 8 gm	**Sodium:** 290 mg
Fat: 4 gm	**Cholesterol:** 5 mg

INGREDIENTS:

2 teaspoons unflavored gelatin

2 tablespoons cold water

Sugar substitute to equal ⅓ cup sugar*

2½ cups 1% low-fat cottage cheese

1 teaspoon vanilla extract

1 (16-ounce) can cherries in water

2 teaspoons cornstarch

Sugar substitute to equal ¼ cup sugar*

⅛ teaspoon almond extract

6 drops red food coloring (optional)

14 (2½-inch) graham cracker squares, crushed

¼ cup reduced-calorie margarine, melted

Sugar substitute to equal 1 tablespoon sugar*

STEPS IN PREPARATION:

1. Sprinkle gelatin over cold water in a small saucepan; let stand 1 minute. Cook over low heat, stirring constantly, 2 minutes or until gelatin dissolves. Let cool.
2. Add sugar substitute to equal ⅓ cup sugar to cooled gelatin.
3. Combine cottage cheese and vanilla in container of an electric blender; cover and process until smooth. Gradually add gelatin mixture to cottage cheese mixture. Place cottage cheese mixture in a bowl, and chill 10 to 12 minutes or until slightly thickened, stirring occasionally.
4. Drain cherries, reserving liquid. Combine cornstarch and cherry liquid in a small saucepan; stir until smooth. Cook over medium heat, stirring constantly, until cornstarch mixture comes to a boil. Reduce heat, and cook 1 minute. Remove from heat, and stir in cherries.
5. Let cherry mixture cool slightly; add sugar substitute to equal ¼ cup sugar, almond extract, and red food coloring, if desired. Set cherry mixture aside.

6. Combine graham cracker crumbs, melted margarine, and sugar substitute to equal 1 tablespoon sugar. Press crumb mixture firmly into a 9-inch pieplate.
7. Spoon cottage cheese mixture into prepared crust; chill 15 minutes. Top with cherry mixture. Cover and chill at least 8 hours.

Yield: 12 servings

*See the sugar substitution chart on page 354.

Vary this basic cheesecake recipe by using fresh fruit instead of the canned cherry mixture. (The exchange values will remain the same.)

Try topping the cheesecake with 2 kiwifruit, peeled and thinly sliced, and 1 cup sliced fresh strawberries. Brush fruit lightly with ¼ cup melted low-sugar apple jelly.

Or arrange 1 cup thinly sliced fresh peaches and ½ cup fresh raspberries on the cake, and brush with melted low-sugar jelly.

INDIVIDUAL FRUITCAKES

Exchanges: 1 Starch, ½ Fruit, 1 Fat

Serving Size: 1 cake
Carbohydrate: 22 gm
Protein: 2 gm
Fat: 6 gm

Calories: 147
Fiber: 2 gm
Sodium: 201 mg
Cholesterol: 0 mg

INGREDIENTS:

Liquid sugar substitute to
 equal 1½ cups sugar*
½ cup unsweetened orange
 juice
1 cup fresh cranberries,
 finely chopped or 1 cup
 sour cherries in water,
 drained and finely chopped
1 cup raisins
1 cup pecans, finely chopped
1 cup pineapple chunks in
 juice, drained and chopped

3 tablespoons reduced-calorie
 margarine, melted
1 tablespoon grated orange
 rind
1½ cups all-purpose flour
1 teaspoon baking soda
½ teaspoon salt
¼ teaspoon ground allspice
¼ teaspoon ground cinnamon
¼ teaspoon ground nutmeg
Vegetable cooking spray

STEPS IN PREPARATION:

1. Pour sugar substitute and orange juice over chopped cranberries;
 let stand 1 hour.
2. Add raisins, pecans, pineapple, margarine, and orange rind to
 cranberry mixture.
3. Combine flour and next 5 ingredients; add dry ingredients to fruit
 mixture, and stir until well blended.
4. Spoon mixture into 16 muffin cups coated with cooking spray.
 Bake at 325° for 30 to 35 minutes or until lightly browned.

Yield: 16 individual cakes

*See the sugar substitution chart on page 354.

RAISIN CAKE

Exchanges: 2 Starch, 1 Fat

Serving Size: 1 slice
Carbohydrate: 37 gm
Protein: 4 gm
Fat: 4 gm

Calories: 197
Fiber: 1 gm
Sodium: 177 mg
Cholesterol: 15 mg

INGREDIENTS:

2 cups water
1 cup reduced-calorie
   margarine
1 (15-ounce) package raisins
Sugar substitute to equal 1
   cup sugar*
2 teaspoons baking soda
¼ cup warm water

2 eggs, lightly beaten
4½ cups all-purpose flour
½ teaspoon baking powder
1 teaspoon ground cloves
1 teaspoon ground allspice
1 teaspoon ground cinnamon
Vegetable cooking spray

STEPS IN PREPARATION:

1. Bring 2 cups water to a boil in a large saucepan; stir in margarine
   and raisins. Let stand, uncovered, 5 minutes. Let raisin mixture
   cool. Stir in sugar substitute.
2. Dissolve soda in ¼ cup warm water; add to raisin mixture, stirring
   well. Stir in eggs.
3. Combine flour and next 4 ingredients; gradually add to raisin
   mixture, stirring after each addition.
4. Spoon batter into a 10-inch Bundt pan coated with cooking spray.
   Bake at 350° for 50 minutes to 1 hour or until a wooden pick
   inserted in center comes out clean. Cool cake in pan 10 minutes.
   Remove from pan; let cool on a wire rack.

Yield: 24 servings

*See the sugar substitution chart on page 354.

ORANGE STREUSEL CAKE

Exchanges: 1½ Starch, ½ Fat

Serving Size: 1 slice
Carbohydrate: 25 gm
Protein: 4 gm
Fat: 3 gm

Calories: 147
Fiber: 1 gm
Sodium: 167 mg
Cholesterol: 15 mg

INGREDIENTS:

1 package dry yeast
Sugar substitute to equal ⅓
   cup sugar, divided*
½ cup warm water (105° to
   115°)
1 egg
2¾ cups all-purpose flour,
   divided
2 tablespoons reduced-calorie
   margarine, melted

2 tablespoons low-sugar
   orange marmalade
½ teaspoon salt
Vegetable cooking spray
¼ cup reduced-calorie
   margarine, melted
1 tablespoon grated orange
   rind
1 tablespoon unsweetened
   orange juice

STEPS IN PREPARATION:

1. Dissolve yeast and one-fifth of sugar substitute in water; let stand
   5 minutes. Add egg, beating well.
2. Add 1 cup flour and next 3 ingredients. Beat until smooth. Add
   1¼ cups flour to make a soft dough.
3. Turn dough out onto a lightly floured surface; knead until smooth
   and elastic. Place in a bowl coated with cooking spray, turning to
   grease top.
4. Cover and let rise in a warm place (85°), free from drafts, 50
   minutes or until doubled in bulk. Punch down. Press into a 9-inch
   round pan coated with cooking spray.
5. Combine remaining sugar substitute, remaining ½ cup flour, ¼
   cup margarine, orange rind, and juice; stir well, and sprinkle over
   dough. Cover and let rise in a warm place, free from drafts, 25
   minutes or until doubled in bulk. Bake at 375° for 25 minutes.

Yield: 12 servings

*See the sugar substitution chart on page 354.

TASTY PINEAPPLE CAKE

Exchanges: 1½ Starch, 1 Fat

Serving Size: 1 slice
Carbohydrate: 26 gm
Protein: 3 gm
Fat: 5 gm

Calories: 158
Fiber: 1 gm
Sodium: 219 mg
Cholesterol: 31 mg

INGREDIENTS:

½ cup reduced-calorie
  margarine
Sugar substitute to equal 2¼
  cups sugar*
2 eggs
1½ cups all-purpose flour
1 teaspoon baking powder

½ teaspoon baking soda
¼ teaspoon salt
½ cup skim milk
4 slices canned pineapple in
  juice, drained
1 tablespoon all-purpose flour
Vegetable cooking spray

STEPS IN PREPARATION:

1. Beat margarine at medium speed of an electric mixer until creamy; gradually add sugar substitute, beating well. Add eggs, one at a time, beating well.
2. Combine 1½ cups flour, baking powder, soda, and salt. Add to creamed mixture alternately with milk, beginning and ending with flour mixture. Beat at low speed after each addition. Cut pineapple into ½-inch pieces; toss with 1 tablespoon flour, and gently fold into batter.
3. Spoon batter into a 6-cup Bundt pan coated with cooking spray. Bake at 350° for 35 to 40 minutes or until a wooden pick inserted in center comes out clean.
4. Remove cake from oven; let stand 5 minutes. Remove cake from pan, and cool completely on a wire rack.

Yield: 12 servings

*See the sugar substitution chart on page 354.

ALMOND COOKIES

Exchanges: ½ Starch

Serving Size: 1 cookie	**Calories:** 51
Carbohydrate: 7 gm	**Fiber:** trace
Protein: 1 gm	**Sodium:** 68 mg
Fat: 2 gm	**Cholesterol:** 13 mg

INGREDIENTS:

¼ cup plus 2 tablespoons
  reduced-calorie margarine
Sugar substitute to equal ¼
  cup sugar*
1 egg yolk
½ teaspoon almond extract

¼ teaspoon vanilla extract
¼ teaspoon lemon extract
1 cup all-purpose flour
½ teaspoon baking powder
⅛ teaspoon salt

STEPS IN PREPARATION:

1. Beat margarine at medium speed of an electric mixer until creamy; gradually add sugar substitute, beating well. Add egg yolk and extracts; beat well.
2. Combine flour, baking powder, and salt; add to creamed mixture, beating well.
3. Shape dough into 1-inch balls; place 2 inches apart on nonstick cookie sheets. Press each with a fork to flatten.
4. Bake at 300° for 20 minutes or until edges begin to brown. Remove cookies to wire racks, and let cool completely.

Yield: 15 cookies

*See the sugar substitution chart on page 354.

APPLESAUCE COOKIES

Exchanges: 1 Starch, ½ Fat

Serving Size: 2 cookies
Carbohydrate: 15 gm
Protein: 2 gm
Fat: 3 gm

Calories: 87
Fiber: 2 gm
Sodium: 208 mg
Cholesterol: 10 mg

INGREDIENTS:

1¾ cups sifted cake flour
1 teaspoon baking soda
½ teaspoon salt
1 teaspoon ground cinnamon
½ teaspoon ground nutmeg
½ teaspoon ground cloves
½ cup reduced-calorie
   margarine

Liquid sugar substitute to
   equal ½ cup sugar*
1 teaspoon vanilla extract
1 egg
1 cup unsweetened
   applesauce
1 cup wheat bran cereal
⅓ cup raisins

STEPS IN PREPARATION:

1. Sift together first 6 ingredients.
2. Combine margarine, sugar substitute, vanilla, and egg; beat well.
3. Add flour mixture and applesauce alternately to creamed mixture, beating well after each addition. Fold in bran cereal and raisins.
4. Drop cookie dough by level tablespoonfuls, 1 inch apart, onto nonstick cookie sheets.
5. Bake at 375° for 10 to 12 minutes or until lightly browned. Remove to wire racks, and let cool completely.

Yield: 3 dozen cookies

*See the sugar substitution chart on page 354.

CINNAMON COOKIES

Exchanges: ½ Starch

Serving Size: 3 cookies	**Calories:** 73
Carbohydrate: 10 gm	**Fiber:** 1 gm
Protein: 1 gm	**Sodium:** 98 mg
Fat: 3 gm	**Cholesterol:** 0 mg

INGREDIENTS:

1 cup all-purpose flour
¼ teaspoon baking powder
¼ cup plus 1 tablespoon
   reduced-calorie margarine
2 teaspoons vanilla extract

Liquid sugar substitute to
   equal ⅓ cup sugar*
1 tablespoon unsweetened
   orange juice
1 teaspoon ground cinnamon

STEPS IN PREPARATION:

1. Combine flour and baking powder in a medium bowl.
2. Combine margarine and vanilla; beat well. Add flour mixture to creamed mixture.
3. Combine sugar substitute and orange juice. Add juice mixture to flour mixture, stirring well.
4. Sprinkle cinnamon over dough, and knead to make a streaked appearance. Shape dough into 30 (½-inch) balls; place on nonstick cookie sheets. Flatten balls with a fork dipped in cold water.
5. Bake at 350° for 12 to 15 minutes or until lightly browned. Remove to wire racks, and let cool completely.

Yield: 2½ dozen cookies

*See the sugar substitution chart on page 354.

LEMON-COCONUT COOKIES

Exchanges: 1 Starch, 1 Fat

Serving Size: 3 cookies
Carbohydrate: 12 gm
Protein: 2 gm
Fat: 4 gm

Calories: 94
Fiber: 1 gm
Sodium: 162 mg
Cholesterol: 10 mg

INGREDIENTS:

½ cup reduced-calorie margarine
Liquid sugar substitute to equal ½ cup sugar*
1 tablespoon water
1 tablespoon grated lemon rind
1 tablespoon lemon juice

1 teaspoon vanilla extract
1 egg
½ cup unsweetened shredded coconut
2 cups all-purpose flour
1 teaspoon baking powder
½ teaspoon salt

STEPS IN PREPARATION:

1. Beat margarine at medium speed of an electric mixer until creamy; gradually add sugar substitute, beating well.
2. Add water and next 4 ingredients; beat until well blended. Add coconut, stirring well.
3. Combine flour, baking powder, and salt. Add to creamed mixture, beating well at low speed.
4. Shape dough into a 2-inch diameter roll; wrap in wax paper. Chill until firm. Cut into 54 thin slices, and place on nonstick cookie sheets.
5. Bake at 375° for 10 to 12 minutes or until lightly browned. Remove to wire racks, and let cool completely.

Yield: 4½ dozen cookies

*See the sugar substitution chart on page 354.

OATMEAL COOKIES

Exchanges: ½ Starch, ½ Fat

Serving Size: 2 cookies	**Calories:** 80
Carbohydrate: 11 gm	**Fiber:** 1 gm
Protein: 2 gm	**Sodium:** 114 mg
Fat: 3 gm	**Cholesterol:** 0 mg

INGREDIENTS:

1½ cups all-purpose flour
½ teaspoon baking soda
¼ teaspoon salt
1½ cups quick-cooking oats, uncooked

Sugar substitute to equal ½ cup sugar*
¾ cup reduced-calorie margarine, softened
3 tablespoons cold water

STEPS IN PREPARATION:

1. Combine first 5 ingredients in a large bowl. Cut margarine into dry mixture with a pastry blender until mixture resembles coarse meal. Sprinkle cold water evenly over surface; stir with a fork until dry ingredients are moistened.
2. Roll dough to ¼-inch thickness on wax paper. Cut into 46 rounds with a 1-inch cookie cutter. Place cookies on nonstick cookie sheets.
3. Bake at 375° for 12 minutes or until lightly browned. Remove to wire racks, and let cool completely.

Yield: 46 cookies

*See the sugar substitution chart on page 354.

SPICED OATMEAL COOKIES

Exchanges: ½ Starch, ½ Fat

Serving Size: 2 cookies
Carbohydrate: 7 gm
Protein: 2 gm
Fat: 3 gm

Calories: 72
Fiber: 1 gm
Sodium: 140 mg
Cholesterol: 16 mg

INGREDIENTS:

1½ cups quick-cooking oats, uncooked
1 cup reduced-calorie margarine, melted
Liquid sugar substitute to equal 1¼ cups sugar*
3 eggs, lightly beaten
1 teaspoon vanilla extract
1¼ cups all-purpose flour

2 teaspoons baking powder
½ teaspoon salt
1 teaspoon ground cinnamon
1 teaspoon ground cloves
1 teaspoon ground nutmeg
½ cup skim milk
¼ cup raisins

STEPS IN PREPARATION:

1. Combine oats and margarine in a large bowl; stir well. Add sugar substitute, eggs, and vanilla; stir until well blended.
2. Combine flour and next 5 ingredients.
3. Add dry ingredients and milk alternately to oatmeal mixture; stir well. Stir in raisins.
4. Drop dough by level teaspoonfuls onto nonstick cookie sheets.
5. Bake at 400° for 10 to 15 minutes or until lightly browned. Remove to wire racks, and let cool completely.

Yield: 6 dozen cookies

*See the sugar substitution chart on page 354.

DATE-OAT BARS

Exchanges: 1 Starch, 1 Fat

Serving Size: 1 bar
Carbohydrate: 14 gm
Protein: 2 gm
Fat: 4 gm

Calories: 95
Fiber: 2 gm
Sodium: 48 mg
Cholesterol: 0 mg

INGREDIENTS:

1 (8-ounce) package pitted dates, chopped
1 tablespoon all-purpose flour
½ cup water
¾ cup unsweetened shredded coconut
½ cup reduced-calorie margarine
Sugar substitute to equal ½ cup sugar*
2½ cups quick-cooking oats, uncooked
½ teaspoon vanilla extract
Vegetable cooking spray

STEPS IN PREPARATION:

1. Combine chopped dates and flour in a large bowl. Toss lightly to coat.
2. Place water in a 1-cup glass measure; microwave at HIGH for 2 to 3 minutes or until boiling. Pour water over dates.
3. Add coconut, margarine, and sugar substitute to date mixture, stirring well. Microwave at HIGH for 2 to 3 minutes or until thickened, stirring at 1-minute intervals. Add oats and vanilla to date mixture, stirring well.
4. Spoon mixture into a 9-inch square pan coated with cooking spray; press evenly into bottom of pan. Cover and chill.
5. Cut into 24 bars, and store in an airtight container in refrigerator.

Yield: 2 dozen bars

*See the sugar substitution chart on page 354.

GRAPE FRAPPÉ

Exchanges: 1 Fruit

Serving Size: 1 cup
Carbohydrate: 17 gm
Protein: 1 gm
Fat: trace

Calories: 91
Fiber: 0 gm
Sodium: 10 mg
Cholesterol: 0 mg

INGREDIENTS:

2⅓ cups water
Sugar substitute to equal 1
  cup sugar*

1 cup unsweetened grape
  juice
Juice of 2 fresh limes

STEPS IN PREPARATION:

1. Combine all ingredients in a medium bowl; stir well. Pour into a freezer tray, and freeze until almost firm.
2. Transfer to a chilled bowl.
3. Beat until fluffy and light in color. Spoon evenly into 4 individual dessert dishes, and serve immediately.

Yield: 4 servings

*See the sugar substitution chart on page 354.

PINEAPPLE SHERBET

Exchanges: ½ Fruit, ½ Whole Milk

Serving Size: ½ cup
Carbohydrate: 15 gm
Protein: 4 gm
Fat: 4 gm

Calories: 110
Fiber: 0 gm
Sodium: 194 mg
Cholesterol: 11 mg

INGREDIENTS:

½ cup half-and-half
Sugar substitute to equal 3
   tablespoons sugar*
1⅓ cups unsweetened
   pineapple juice

4 egg whites
¼ teaspoon salt

STEPS IN PREPARATION:

1. Combine half-and-half and sugar substitute, and freeze.
2. Freeze pineapple juice separately.
3. Combine frozen pineapple juice and frozen half-and-half mixture; beat until smooth.
4. Beat egg whites and salt until stiff peaks form. Fold beaten egg whites into pineapple juice mixture; freeze until firm. To serve, scoop mixture evenly into 4 individual dessert dishes.

Yield: 4 servings

*See the sugar substitution chart on page 354.

VANILLA ICE CREAM

Exchanges: ½ Skim Milk, 1 Fat

Serving Size: ½ cup
Carbohydrate: 7 gm
Protein: 5 gm
Fat: 6 gm

Calories: 102
Fiber: 0 gm
Sodium: 151 mg
Cholesterol: 78 mg

INGREDIENTS:

1 tablespoon unflavored gelatin
1¼ cups skim milk, divided
2 eggs, separated
¼ teaspoon salt

Sugar substitute to equal ¼ cup sugar*
1 cup half-and-half
2 teaspoons vanilla extract

STEPS IN PREPARATION:

1. Soften gelatin in ¼ cup milk; set aside.
2. Combine remaining 1 cup milk, egg yolks, and salt in a double boiler; heat until mixture coats spoon. Remove from heat.
3. Add gelatin mixture and sugar substitute; stir until blended, and let cool. Add half-and-half and vanilla. Freeze until firm.
4. Beat egg whites until stiff peaks form.
5. Remove cream mixture from freezer, and place in a chilled bowl; beat until smooth. Fold in stiffly beaten egg whites. Return to freezer, and freeze until firm.

Yield: 6 servings

*See the sugar substitution chart on page 354.

Sugar Substitutions

Brand Name of Sugar Substitute		Equivalent Amount of Sugar
Adolph's	2 shakes of jar	1 teaspoon sugar
	¼ teaspoon	1 tablespoon sugar
	1 teaspoon	¼ cup sugar
	2½ teaspoons	⅔ cup sugar
	1 tablespoon	¾ cup sugar
	4 teaspoons	1 cup sugar
Equal*	1 packet	2 teaspoons sugar
NutraSweet Spoonful	1 teaspoon	1 teaspoon sugar
Sugar Twin	1 teaspoon	1 teaspoon sugar
Sugar Twin, Brown	1 teaspoon	1 teaspoon brown sugar
Sweet Magic	1 packet	2 teaspoons sugar
Sweet'ner	1 packet	2 teaspoons sugar
Sweet N' Low	⅒ teaspoon	1 teaspoon sugar
	1 packet	2 teaspoons sugar
	⅓ teaspoon	1 tablespoon sugar
	1½ teaspoons	¼ cup sugar
	1 tablespoon	½ cup sugar
	2 tablespoons	1 cup sugar
Sweet N' Low, Brown	¼ teaspoon	1 tablespoon brown sugar
	1 teaspoon	¼ cup brown sugar
	4 teaspoons	1 cup brown sugar
Sweet One	1 packet	2 teaspoons sugar
	3 packets	¼ cup sugar
	4 packets	⅓ cup sugar
	6 packets	½ cup sugar
	12 packets	1 cup sugar

Fasweet (liquid)	⅛ teaspoon	1 teaspoon sugar
	¼ teaspoon	2 teaspoons sugar
	⅓ teaspoon	1 tablespoon sugar
	1 tablespoon	½ cup sugar
	2 tablespoons	1 cup sugar
Sucaryl (liquid)	⅛ teaspoon	1 teaspoon sugar
	⅓ teaspoon	1 tablespoon sugar
	½ teaspoon	4 teaspoons sugar
	1½ teaspoons	¼ cup sugar
	1 tablespoon	½ cup sugar
Superose (liquid)	4 drops	1 teaspoon sugar
	⅛ teaspoon	2 teaspoons sugar
	¼ teaspoon	1 tablespoon sugar
	1½ teaspoons	½ cup sugar
	1 tablespoon	1 cup sugar
Sweet-10 (liquid)	10 drops	1 teaspoon sugar
	½ teaspoon	4 teaspoons sugar
	1½ teaspoons	¼ cup sugar
	1 tablespoon	½ cup sugar
	2 tablespoons	1 cup sugar
Zero-Cal (liquid)	10 drops	1 teaspoon sugar
	30 drops	1 tablespoon sugar
	¾ teaspoon	2 tablespoons sugar
	1 tablespoon	½ cup sugar
	2 tablespoons	1 cup sugar

Note: Sugar equivalents for various brand names of sugar substitutes are listed for your convenience and are not an endorsement of any product.

*Use only after cooking or in uncooked dishes.

Recipe Index

Subject Index

ACKNOWLEDGMENTS

Oxmoor House gratefully acknowledges the contribution of the following people who have helped to make this cookbook possible:

Charlotte Knight Beeker

Mandy Berry

Sandra Dillon, M.A., R.D.

Lynn Epps Eden, M.S., R.D.

Yolanda Guyton

Linda Harbour, R.D.

Susan Hommerson, M.S., R.D.

Sarah Hood, M.S., R.D.

Elizabeth Ivins

Margaret Stewart McDonald, R.D.

Cassandra C. Mills

Laura Moore

Lisa Mullins, M.S., R.D.

Kimberly Garrison Nunn

Margaret Palmer, M.S., R.D.

Bessie Rawls

Debra Simerly, M.S., R.D.

Cynthia Wren